Happiness is when what you think, say + do
are in harmony.

Blendit and mendit.com

Alfredo Sauce

2 c. cashews soaked 30 minutes
1 clove garlic
1/2 of lemon's juice
1 c water
1 t. salt
1 T nutritional yeast flakes

Spiralize zucchini — garnish with basil + tomato.

Veg. Juice

(V5) Kale, 2 tomatoes, yellow pepper, celery, parsley
2 T worstishire sauce, capful Louisiana Hot Sauce
1 1/2 t. salt, 4 ice cubes, 3 c. water

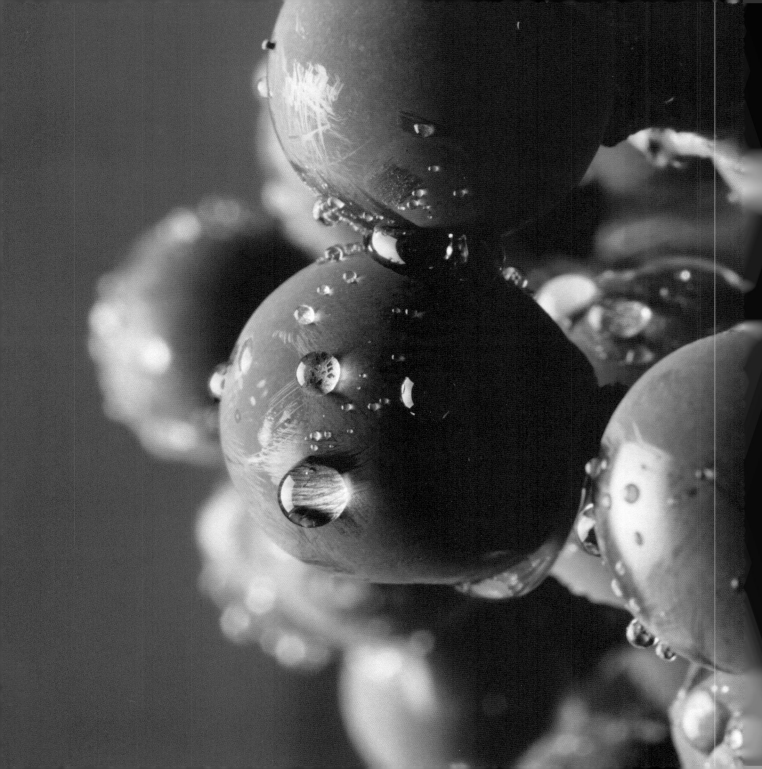

EASY TO BE RAW

Over 30 Simple Recipes To Delight Your Tastebuds On A Daily Basis

By: Megan Elizabeth

EASY TO BE RAW

Over 30 Simple Recipes To Delight Your Tastebuds On A Daily Basis
By: Megan Elizabeth

Photography by Joey Borden, Shaie Dively, Megan Elizabeth McDonnell, Richard McDonnell and Timothy Radley.

Cover design and layout by Joey Borden and Megan Elizabeth McDonnell

Edited by Jim and Mary Borden

DEDICATION

This book is dedicated to everyone who has supported me in my raw food and optimal health seeking journey. Thank you for your encouragement, love and friendship. A special thanks goes to my parents, Patricia Devoy McDonnell and Richard McDonnell, my brother Sean, Joey Borden, Timothy Radley, Arnold Kauffman, and all my friends from Arnold's Way.

"Each of us need all of us and all of us need each of us." - *Jim Rohn*

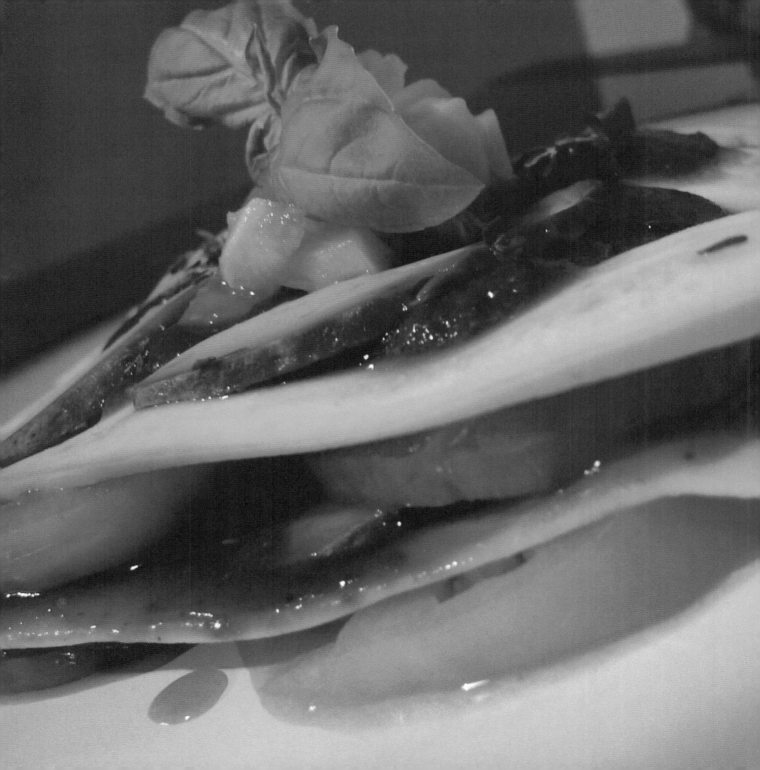

TABLE OF CONTENTS

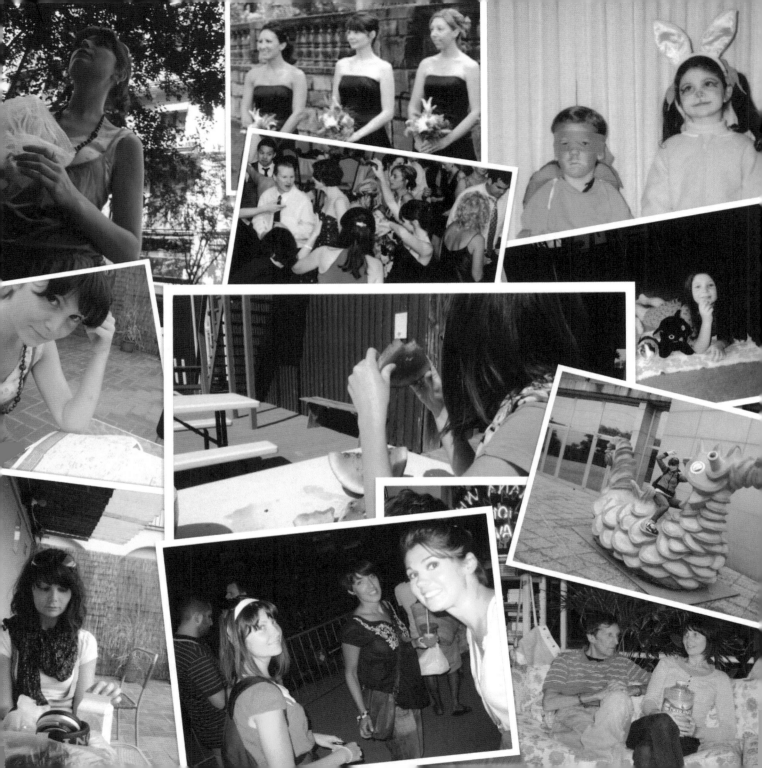

INTRODUCTION
My Story

From the time I can remember choosing what I ate, I was vegetarian. The idea of putting a squishy vein-filled piece of meat in my mouth was simply gross. "How did everyone enjoy this?", I thought. Around age seven or eight I began having adverse effects to dairy products, so I stayed away from that for a while as well. My mom always did her best to make something special for me to eat.

As I approached my teen years I began to try new foods, which included meat. As I experimented with this, I also included dairy occasionally as well. Cheese! I loved cheese! Fat, salt, and addictive casomorphins. What's not to love? I didn't associate any health issues I had, beyond the occasional reactions to dairy, with the food I was eating. I wasn't a particularly sick teenager, but I do remember taking antibiotics often, having extremely imbalanced hormones, and a fluctuating weight problem. I did have a very overweight period at the age of 18 where I maxed out at 170 pounds. "Wow! How did I let myself get to this point?" It must have been all those cosmic brownies.

Approaching twenty I began to refine my diet, including more of what I thought to be healthy foods. I got off dairy again, which resulted in an almost immediate five pound weight loss. I was eating low-carb diet foods, more protein, salads every day, and lots of soy milk! I began exercising regularly and feeling better overall.

Age twenty-one, at 125 pounds, I had reinvented myself and I thought I was looking good. I was a social butterfly, out all night with friends, working and going to college to get my bachelors degree in radiology and MRI. The summer of 2007 I was having more fun than ever. I was kayaking, hiking, swimming, partying a lot, and working a fun, part-time job at a retail doll store with my friend. My summer of low sleep and high activity eventually caught up to me.

At the beginning of my downward spiral was an allergic reaction I had to some make-up in August 2007, right before a road trip to California with my mom. My eyes swelled up and I had horrible headaches. I took a tapered dose of prednisone to help the swelling go down before our trip. On our way out there we barely slept and we made it across the country in three and a half days. I started to feel spacey and mentally exhausted, which I attributed to the lack of sleep and the steroids I had taken.   A week passed since I stopped the steroids and that feeling didn't go away.

I started school again at the end of the month. I found myself unable to concentrate and had constant dull head and neck aches. In the next eight months I experienced the most physical and emotional pain of my life. I became allergic to all chemicals, my hair began to fall out, my skin broke out in rashes and turned grey from malabsorption of nutrients, I dropped down to 108 pounds, and my brain fog was so bad I felt like I was in a dream. It was a nightmare! I had to drop out of school and stop working.

In March 2008 I began to see a holistic doctor who put me on a strict regimen of natural supplement-packed smoothies. I was on a rotation diet to avoid food allergies and switch to all organic food and products. It was like being a sick elderly person; carrying around a huge pill box of supplements. I became slightly more functional and was grateful for that, but I wanted my life back.

A full year passed before my dad discovered "Arnold's Way", an organic raw vegan cafe in Lansdale, Pennsylvania. My dad explained my situation to Arnold Kauffman. He told him how I was eating a very strict organic diet with lots of smoothies and natural supplements. Arnold said to my dad, "I'll destroy that!". My dad told me he found an organic cafe, which sparked my attention since I could no longer go out to eat, and that I needed to speak to the owner who was some kind of health guru.

I went to Arnold's Way for the first time near the end of August 2008 and I have been in almost every day since then. I worked there for a period of time learning as much as I could and developing a new set of skills in preparing raw food. I spent a period of time at first transitioning with high-fat gourmet raw food; however this did not give me the results I was looking for. Although I saw a slight improvement, it was not until I began to follow "natural hygiene" that I saw a huge health turnaround. I discovered a whole new world of fruit besides the typical ones we see in the grocery store. Mangos, durian, jackfruit, and sapodillas are my favorites. I have found that the simplest form of the raw diet is what works for me. Eating lots of whole fresh fruits and vegetables has given me back my health and my life.

Through my own experience I have gained so much passion and knowledge about creating and maintaining a healthy body. I hope to help others prevent illness and achieve their health and fitness goals through sharing what I have learned. Everyone must take responsibility for their own health .

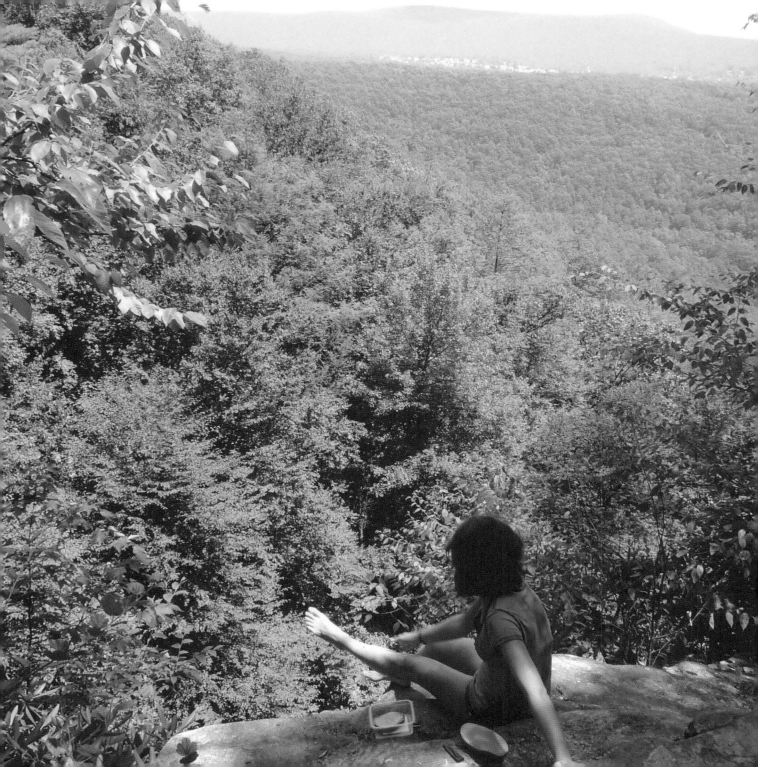

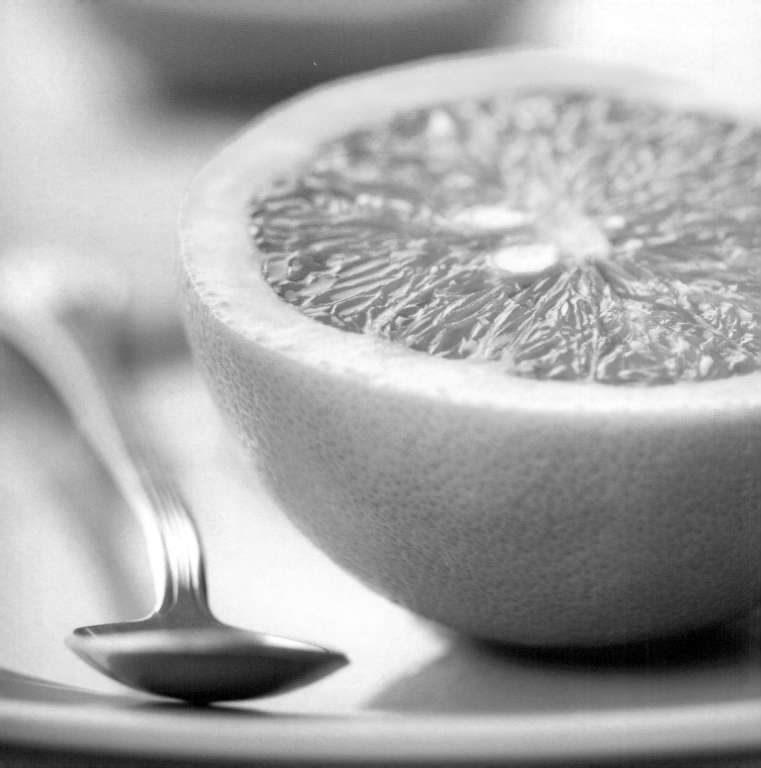

INTRODUCTION
Raw Food

The raw food diet may seem complicated at first and you may think you need expensive equipment to make healthy food. If this was true, fruit would not be so delicious and easy to eat. The recipes in this book are simple and fresh. There is no need to dehydrate or over process food to create amazing taste.

These recipes are also 100% vegan.   Following a raw vegan diet has made me more conscious about the effects my food choices have on my body and our planet. We do not need to use other animals to delight our taste buds. Bees make honey for bees not humans.

Our bodies are naturally in a state of health and unnaturally in a state of disease or sickness. When we remove the cause rather than cover the symptoms, we are moving towards better health.

TAKING RAW WITH YOU
6 Tips for Sticking To It

1. Educate Yourself - Read as much as you need to feel confident about following a raw or vegan diet.

2. Make New Friends - Meet new people who support your lifestyle, so you will not feel alienated for being different. Check your area or local raw cafe/health food store for potlucks and meet-ups. You can also sign up with one of the many raw food forums online. There are plenty of fish in the sea (for now).

3. Don't Let Yourself Get Too Hungry - Having an empty stomach or low blood sugar can cause you to make poor food choices you may regret later.

4. Remember How Easy it Can Be - You *can* have just fruit for dinner. You do not need to have an elaborate meal to feel satisfied. Mono-meals can be the most satisfying of all.

5. Always Take Food With You - If you are going to be out all day, take a six pack with you, a six pack of bananas that is. You can also make one or two smoothies to take with you.

6. Fruit is Ready and Waiting, Wherever You Are - Every grocery store has fruit. Every country has grocery stores. Many stores are starting to carry more organic fruits and vegetables so the options are only growing.

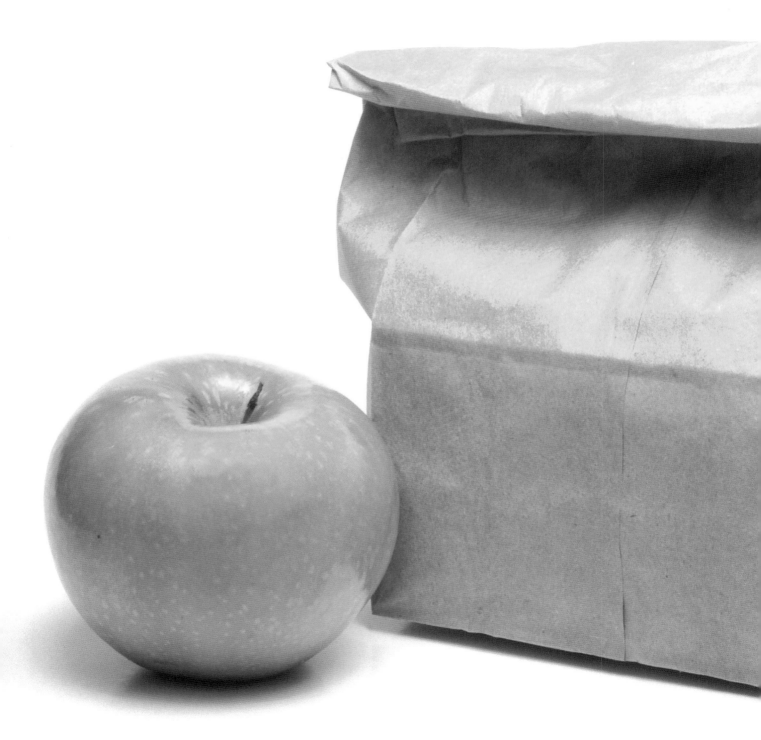

IS THIS THING RIPE?
Eating Ripe Fruit is Important

There are many different ways to tell when fruit is ripe. Often it will have a sweet smell like a mango or an aromatic smell like an heirloom tomato. Many fruits need to be soft as well. An avocado is a good example of a fruit that must be soft, but does not have an aroma. There are some some fruits that change color when they are ripe. Payayas and bananas turn from green to yellow. It is important to eat fruit when it is ripe because eating unripe fruit can cause indigestion. Nutrients and taste are at their peak during ripeness. If you are looking to try a new fruit do a little research first to find out when it is in season and how to tell when it is ripe. Enjoying the taste of a perfectly ripe mango will never get boring to me.

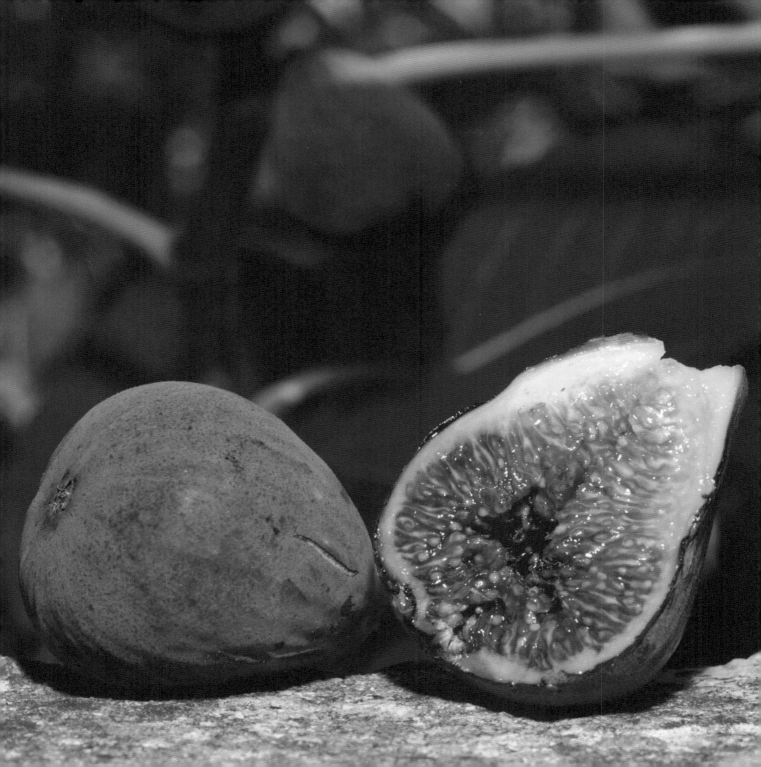

EQUIPMENT REQUIRED

Blender

For almost every recipe in this book you will need a blender. I recommend a Vita-Mix Blender, which is what I use. If you already have another home blender that you can use, that is fine. Make sure to chop the ingredients into small enough pieces for the type of blender you are using.

Food Processor

A few of the recipes in this book call for a food processor. The brand that I recommend is Cuisinart. They are durable, easy to use, and come in a wide range of prices and sizes.

Spiral Slicer

A couple of the recipes in this book call for a spiral slicer. There are many brands available online that are reasonably priced. It is definitely worth the small investment long-term. I use mine a few times a week.

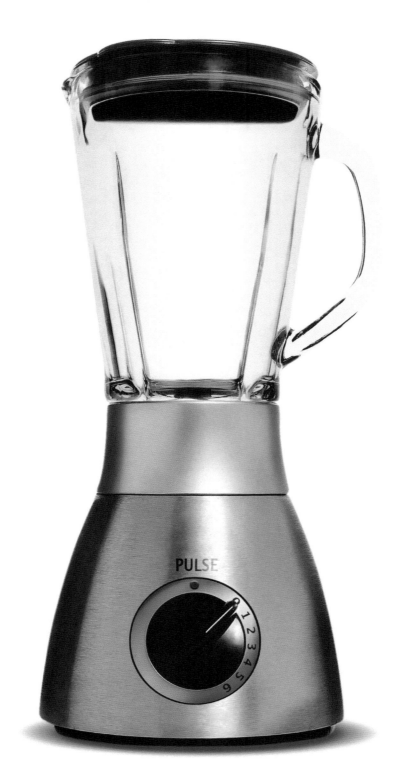

SOUPS

Raw soups are quick and easy to make. They go great with salads or can stand on their own. They can be refreshing in the summer, like papaya gazpacho, or comforting in the winter, like the zucchini noodle with a little extra avocado. Once you learn how to make a good soup base you can experiment with different ingredients.

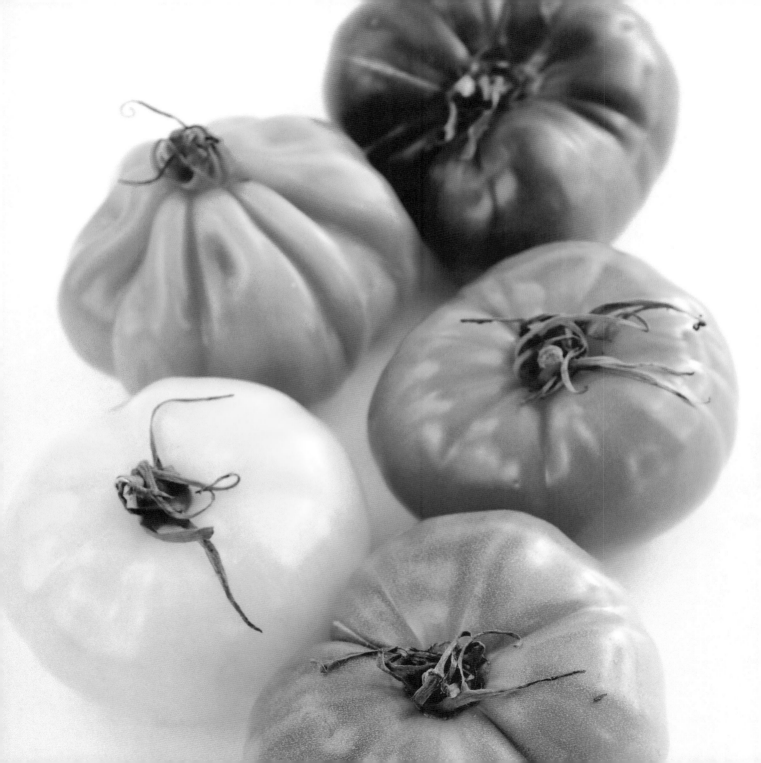

CORN CHOWDER

Ingredients

2 1/2 Cups Fresh Corn off the Cob
2 Cups Chopped Roma Tomatoes
1 Cup Chopped Mango
1 Cup Chopped Celery
1/8 Cup Fresh Squeezed Lemon Juice
2 Pitted Medjool Dates
1/4 Avocado

Directions

Place 2 cups of fresh corn, 1 1/2 cups of chopped roma tomatoes, 1 cup of chopped celery, 1 cup chopped mango, 1/8 cup fresh squeezed lemon juice, 2 pitted medjool dates and 1/4 of an avocado into the blender and blend until creamy. Pour into a large bowl and add 1/2 cup of corn and 1/2 cup of chopped roma tomatoes. Serves 1 to 2 people.

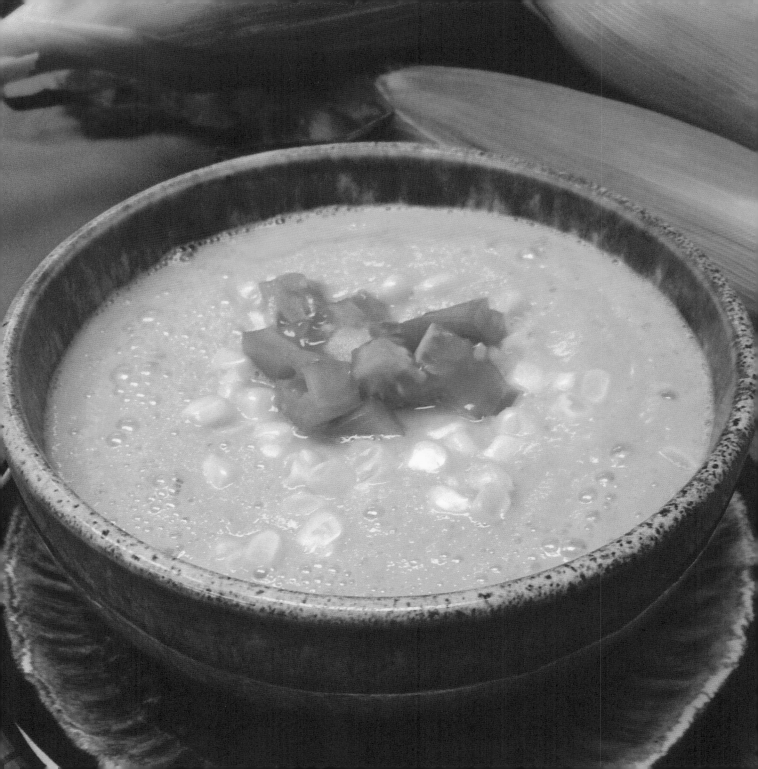

PAPAYA GAZPACHO

Ingredients

2 1/2 Cups Chopped Roma Tomatoes
2 Cups Peeled Chopped Papaya
1 Cup Chopped Celery
1 Cup Peeled Chopped Mango
1/2 Cup Chopped Scallions
2 Quarter-Sized Medallion of Fresh Ginger

Directions

Place 2 cups of peeled chopped papaya, 2 cups chopped roma tomatoes, 1 cup chopped celery, 1 cup peeled chopped mango, 1/2 cup chopped scallions, and 2 quarter-sized medallions of ginger cut into smaller pieces into the blender. Blend until creamy and add ½ cup chopped tomatoes. Serves 1 to 2 people.

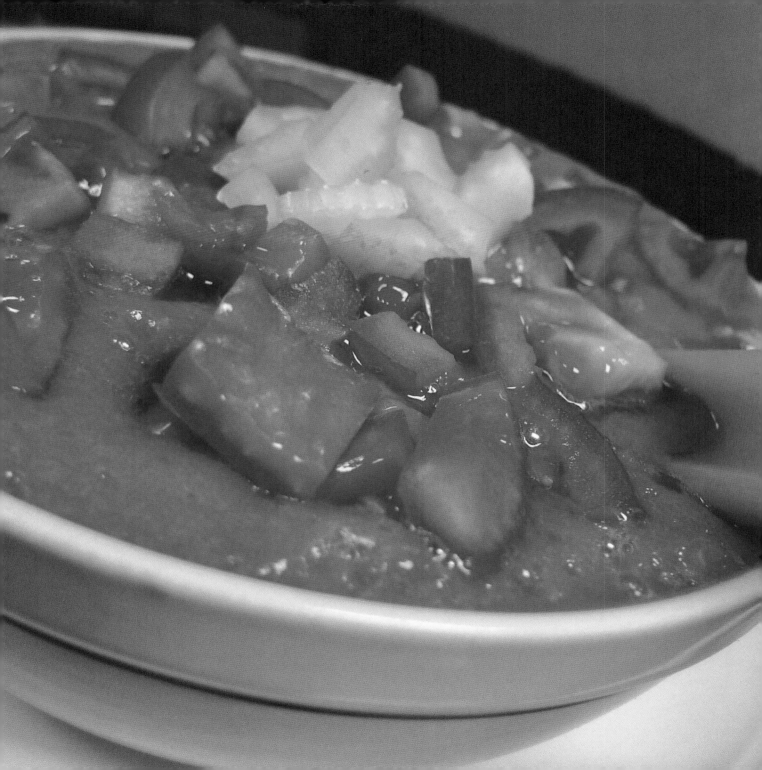

TOMATO CHERRY SOUP

Ingredients

3 1/2 Cups Chopped Roma Tomatoes
2 1/4 Cups Frozen Pre-Pitted Cherries (Mostly or All Thawed)
3 to 4 Medium to Large Leaves of Basil
1 Cup Peeled and Diced Cucumber

Directions

Place 3 cups of chopped roma tomatoes, 2 1/4 cups thawed pre-pitted cherries, and 3 to 4 medium to large leaves of basil into the blender and blend until creamy. Pour into a large bowl and add 1/2 cup chopped roma tomato and 1 cup peeled and diced cucumber to the bowl. Serves 1 to 2 people.

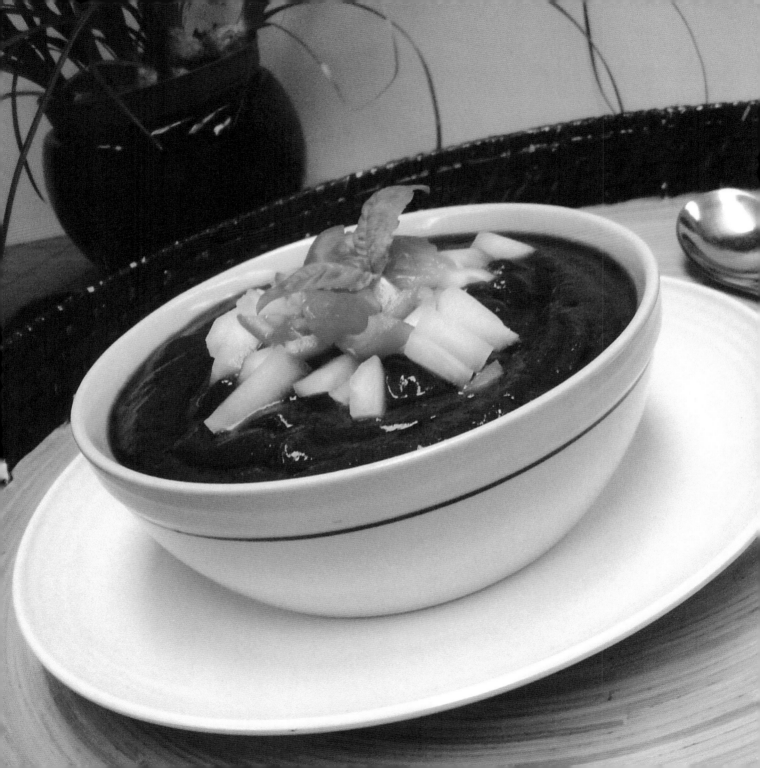

ZUCCHINI NOODLE SOUP

Ingredients

2 Cups Chopped Roma Tomatoes
1 1/2 Cups Fresh Squeezed Orange Juice
1/4 Cup Soaked Sun Dried Tomatoes
1/4 Cup Chopped Red Pepper
2 Pitted Medjool Dates
1/4 Avocado (Optional)
1 1/2 Cups Spiraled Zucchini

Directions

Place 1 1/2 cups of fresh squeezed orange juice, 2 cups chopped roma to-matoes, 1/4 cup soaked sun dried tomatoes, 1/4 cup red pepper, 2 pitted medjool dates, and the optional 1/4 of an avocado into the blender. Blend until creamy. Pour into a large bowl. Spiral 1/2 to 1 whole zucchini to get 1 1/2 cup spiraled zucchini. Cut the zucchini noodles to be about 2 inches in length and add them to the soup. (If you do not own a spiral cutter you can use a simple peeler to make the noodles.) Serves 1 to 2 people.

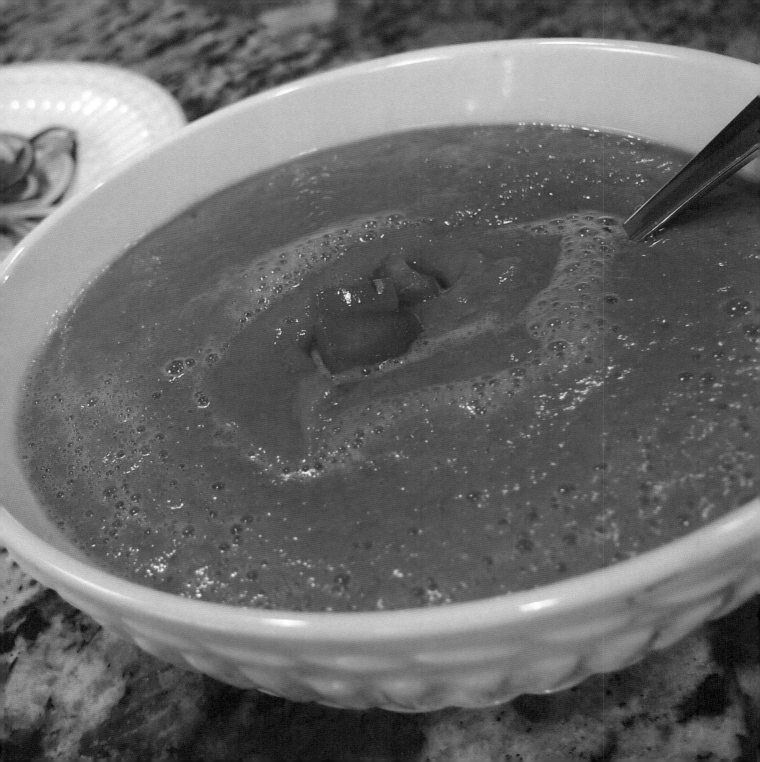

SALADS & DRESSINGS

One of the most common raw salad dressings is olive oil.   How boring is that? Not only is it a refined food, but it is empty calories of pure fat! Eating raw food is not just about not heating food, it is also about eating whole foods. Always try to make your salad out of whole foods. Avocados and dates make great bases for a salad dressing and can be flavored with any other whole food that you like.

Creamy zucchini tomato Alfredo

Spring mix + tomatoes

Dressing:
  2 1/2 T lemon juice
  1/2 c hemp seeds
  3 leaves basil
  1 T Rosemary
  1/2 T thyme
  little bit chopped tomato (for liquid)
  1 T tahini

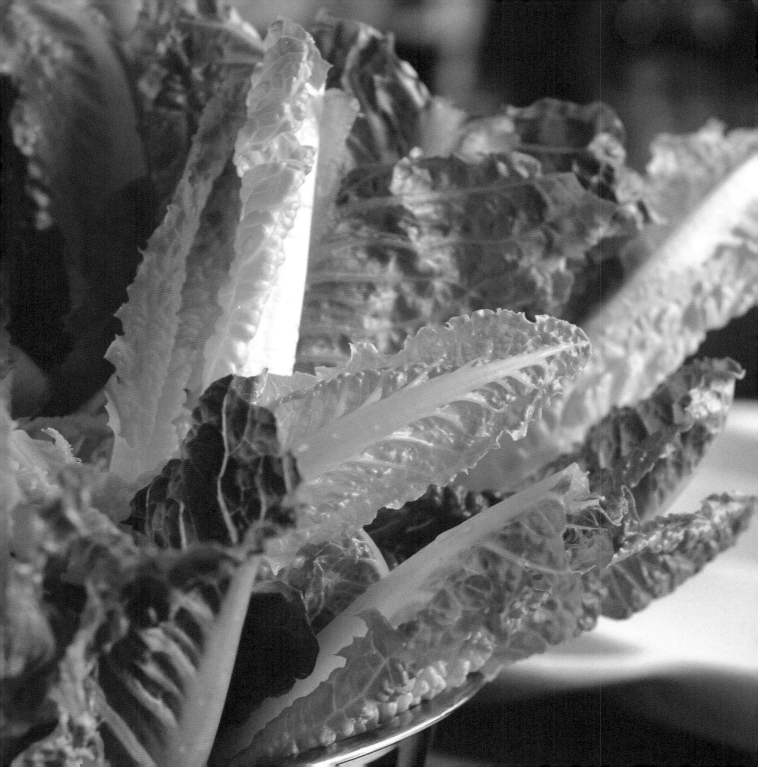

GARDEN HERB SALAD

Ingredients

1 1/2 Cups Chopped Fresh Parsley
1/2 Cup Chopped Fresh Cilantro
1/2 Cup Fresh Squeezed Lemon Juice
4 Pitted Medjool Dates
1/4 Avocado
1 Cup Chopped Apple
1/2 Cup Grapes Chopped in Half
1/2 Cup Chopped Celery
1/8 Cup Shredded Carrot as Garnish
3 Chopped Romaine Hearts

TinaJo
Jicama / apple Salad

Dice J + A
orange pepper
sweet corn
cilantro
green onion

Dressing
(add miso + cumin)
pumpkin seeds on top

Directions

Place 1 1/2 cups chopped fresh parsley, 1/2 cup chopped fresh cilantro, 4 pitted medjool dates, 1/2 cup fresh squeezed lemon and 1/4 of an avocado into the blender. Blend until creamy. Toss 1 cup chopped apple, 1/2 cup grapes chopped in half, 1/2 cup chopped celery, and 3 chopped romaine hearts in a large salad bowl. Pour the dressing on the salad and toss or leave on the side. Garnish the salad with the 1/8 cup shredded carrot. Serves 2 to 4 people.

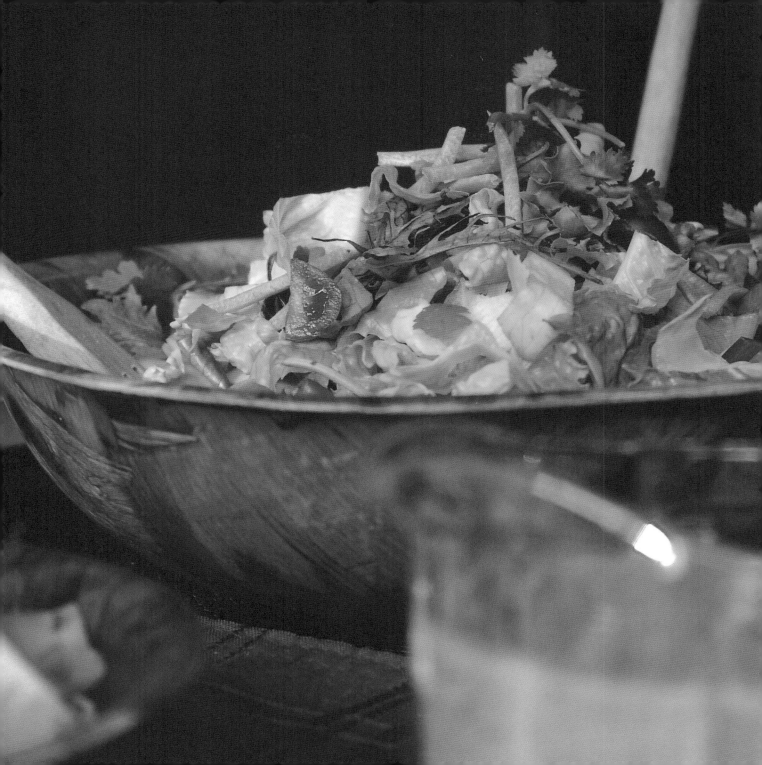

GUACAMOLE SALAD

Ingredients

3/4 Cup Chopped Scallions
3/4 Cup Water
1/2 Cup Fresh Squeezed Lemon Juice
6 to 8 Leaves of Cilantro
4 Pitted Medjool Dates
1/2 Avocado
2 Cups Chopped Roma Tomatoes
1 Cup Fresh Sweet Corn off the Cob
3 Chopped Romaine Hearts

Directions

Place 3/4 cup chopped scallions, 3/4 cup of water, 1/2 cup fresh squeezed lemon, 6 to 8 leaves of cilantro, 4 pitted medjool dates, and 1/2 of an avocado into the blender. Blend until creamy. Toss the 2 cups of chopped roma tomatoes, 1 cup of fresh sweet corn, and 3 chopped romaine hearts in a large bowl. Pour the dressing on the salad and toss or leave on the side. Serves 2 to 4 people.

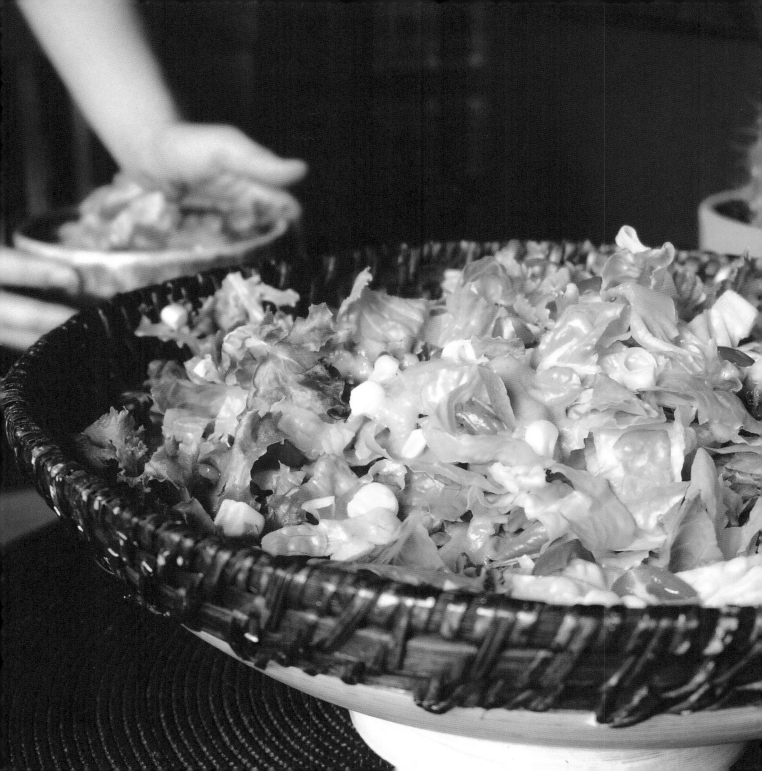

MANGO SUMMER SALAD

Ingredients

2 1/2 Cups Chopped Mango
1/4 to 1/2 Cup Water
1 Teaspoon Finely Ground Cinnamon
4 Pitted Medjool Dates
1 Cup Chopped Apple
1/2 Cup Chopped Roma Tomatoes
1 Tablespoon Shredded Coconut (optional)
3 Chopped Hearts of Romaine

Directions

Place 2 cups of chopped mango, 1/4 cup of water, 1 teaspoon finely ground cinnamon, and 4 pitted medjool dates into the blender. Blend until creamy and add extra water as needed. Toss the 1 cup chopped apple, 1/2 cup of chopped mango, 1/2 cup of chopped roma tomatoes, 3 chopped romaine hearts, and the optional 1 tablespoon shredded coconut in a large salad bowl. Pour the dressing on the salad and toss or leave on the side. Serves 2 to 4 people.

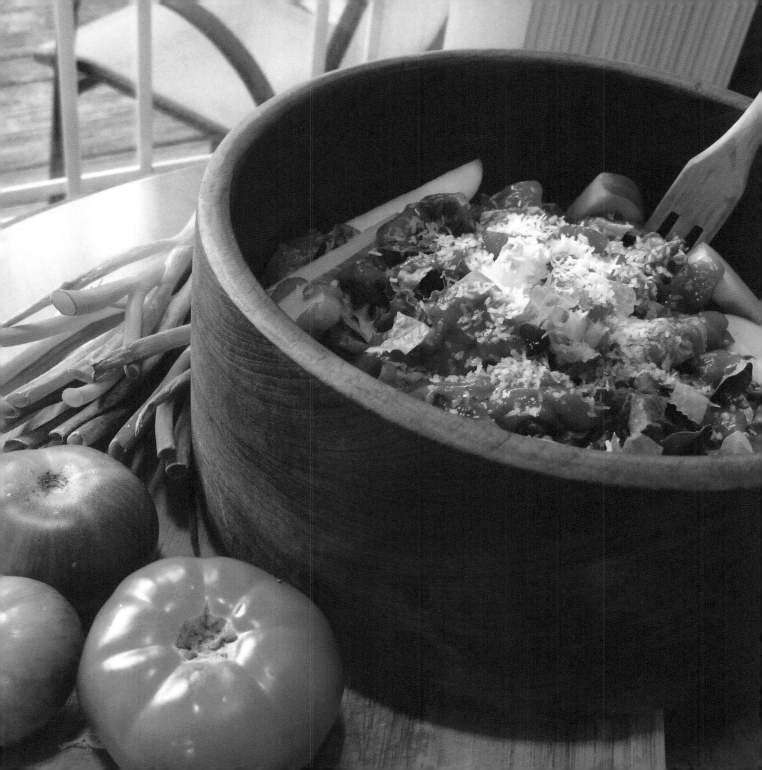

TANGY SCALLION SALAD

Ingredients

2 Cups Chopped Scallions
2 Cups Chopped Mango
1/2 to 2/3 Cup Water
4 Pitted Medjool Dates
1 Cup Chopped Roma Tomatoes
3 Chopped Hearts of Romaine

Directions

Place 1 1/2 cups of chopped mango, 1 cup of chopped scallions, 1/2 cup of water and 4 pitted medjool dates into the blender. Blend until creamy and add extra water as necessary. Toss the 3 chopped romaine hearts, 1 cup of chopped roma tomatoes, 1 cup of chopped scallions and 1/2 cup of chopped mango in a large salad bowl. Pour the dressing on the salad and toss or leave on the side. Serves 2 to 4 people.

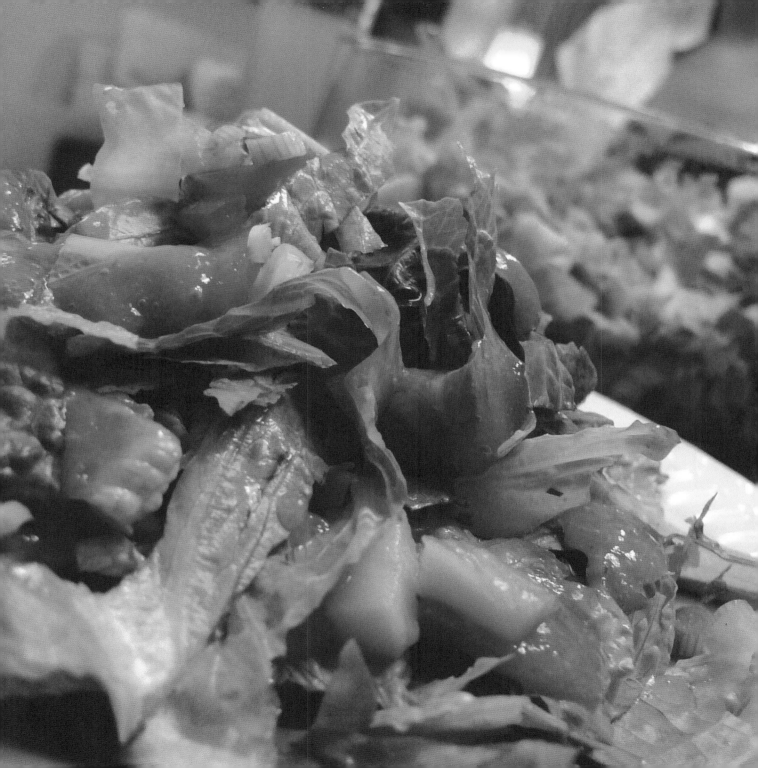

GINGER ORANGE DELIGHT

Ingredients

1/8 Cup Fresh Squeezed Lemon
2 Whole Oranges (or About 2 Cups) Peeled and Chopped
2 Pitted Medjool Dates
1 Quarter Sized Medallion of Fresh Ginger

Make Your Own Salad

This salad dressing will taste great with the mango summer salad or you can create your own salad. Try mixing it up with fruits and vegetables you haven't used before. There are thousands of varieties of fruits and veggies in the world, so you shouldn't have trouble finding something new.

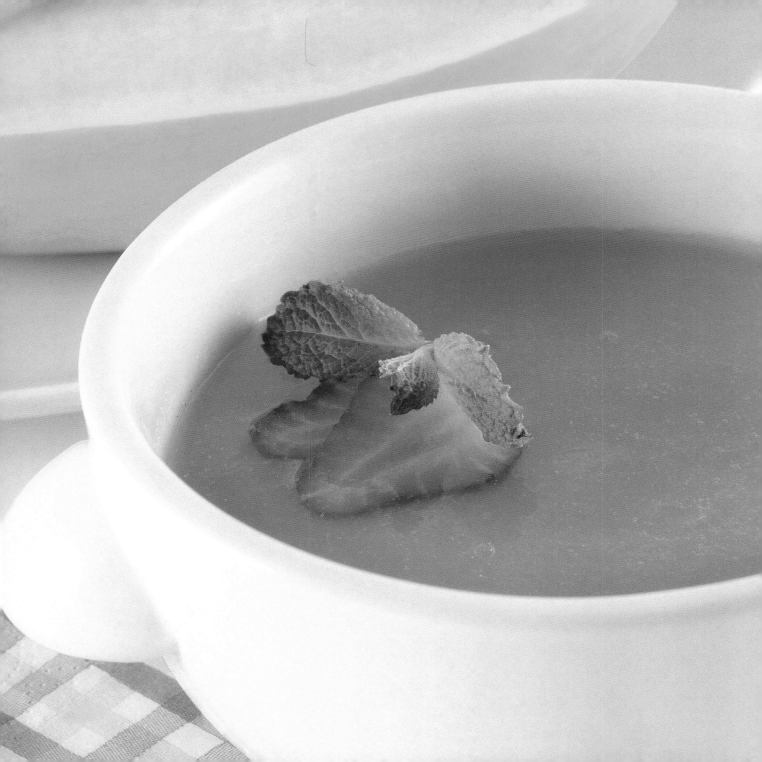

PINK LADY

Ingredients

2 Cups Peeled Chopped Papaya
1/2 Cup Fresh Chopped Strawberries
1/4 Cup Fresh Squeezed Lime Juice
2 Pitted Medjool Dates

Directions

Place all the ingredients in the blender and blend until creamy.

Winning Combo

I'm almost positive the pink ladies and greasers have never tried this dressing, but it sure is pink! Papaya and lime is a winning combination whether on its own, in a smoothie or on top of a salad. This is a sure taste bud pleaser. You can use this dressing with the mango sumer salad (page 30), the tangy scallion salad (page 32), or make up your own.

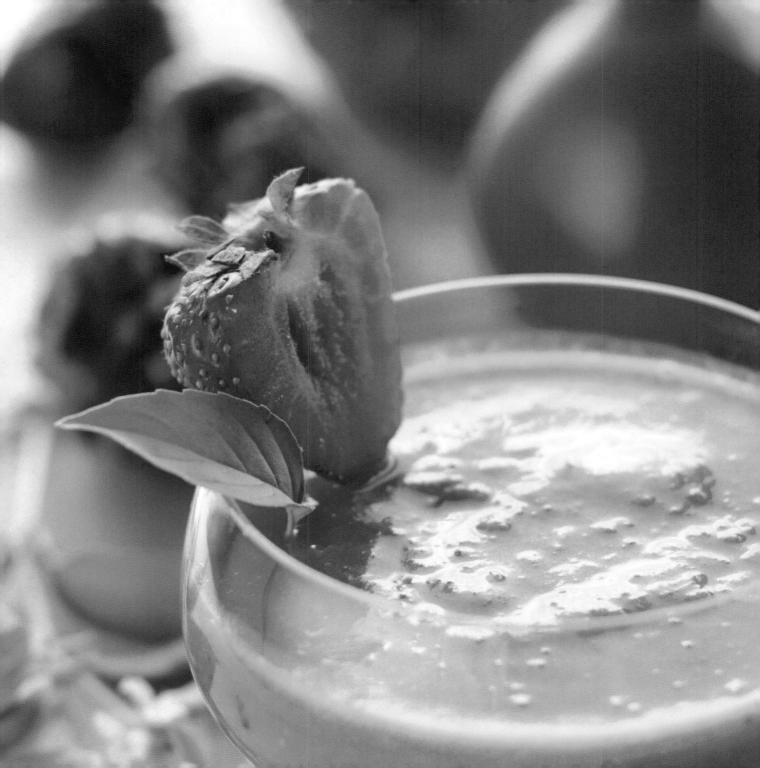

SWEET AND SPICY SESAME

Ingredients

1/4 Cup Water
1/8 Cup Raw Sesame Seeds
1/8 Cup Raw Mustard Seeds
3 Pitted Medjool Dates
2 Whole Oranges (or About 2 Cups) Peeled and Chopped

Directions

Place all the ingredients in the blender and blend until creamy.

Kick it!

This salad dressing has a little kick to it with those mustard seeds. Try making a salad with some asian flare or even a slaw with shredded carrot, raisin, and whatever else you fancy. Also, sesame seeds, used in this dressing, are one of the best non-dairy sources of calcium. They have about 90mg per tablespoon.

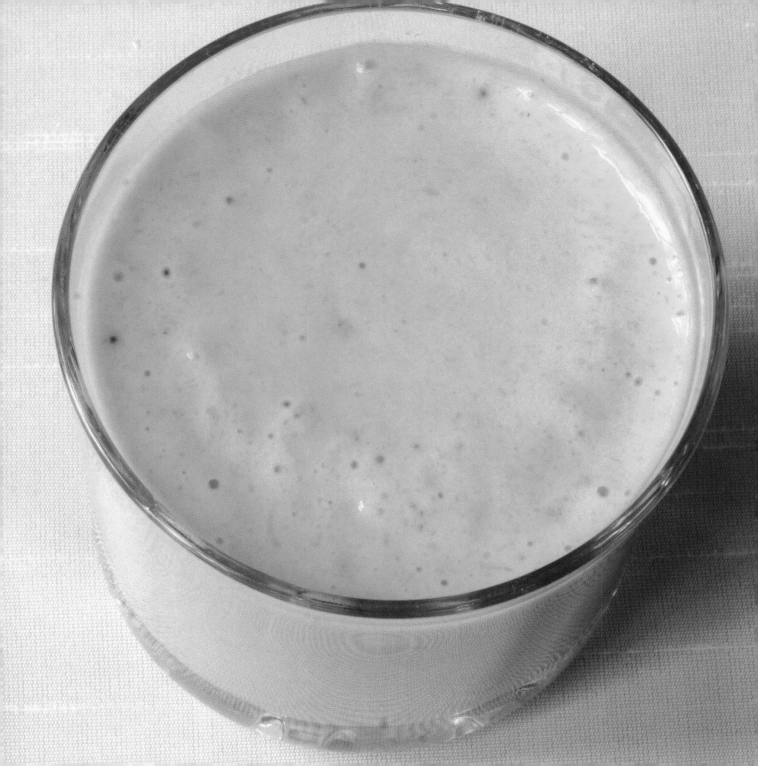

APPETIZERS

Tip number four for sticking to the raw diet is to remember how easy it can be. The appetizers in this book can all be made in 10 minutes or less and contain minimal ingredients. I always encourage experimentation! Most of my recipes can be slightly altered to use seasonal ingredients or add your own touch.

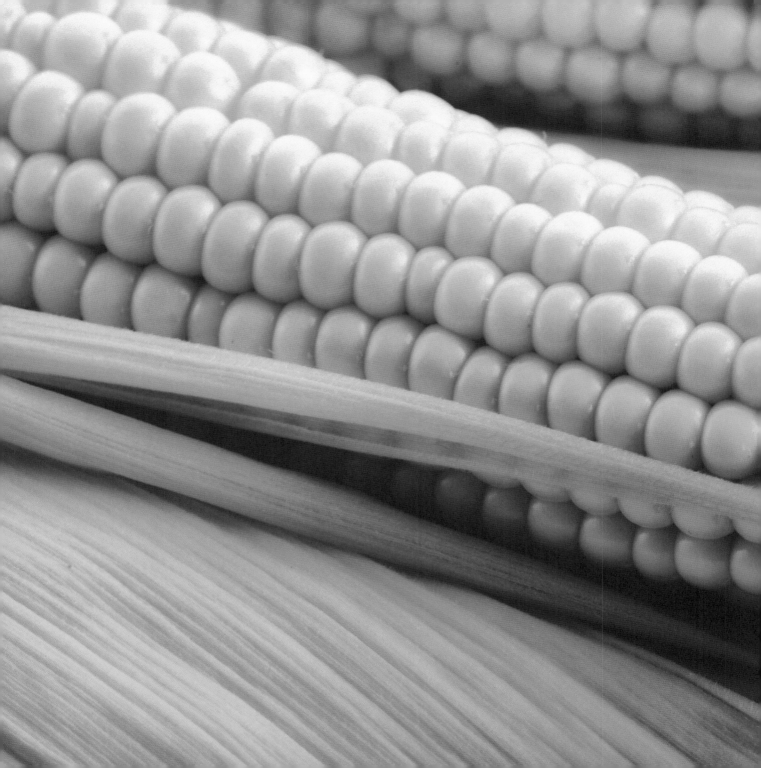

SWEET CORN AND TOMATO SALAD

This super delicious and easy recipe was created during my annual summer vacation in a small town in Ontario, Cananda. We stay on a small island near the mainland. One year, a group of us paddle boated to shore, walked a mile to the nearest farm and bought fresh corn and tomatoes. We used a few things we already had back at the house and created this yummy dish.

Ingredients

3 Cups Fresh Sweet Corn Off the Cobb
2 Cups Chopped Roma Tomatoes
1/2 Cup Chopped Celery — or anything green (cuke, broccoli, dandelion greens etc)
1/8 Cup Fresh Squeezed Lemon Juice (½ lemon)
1/4 Avocado Chopped (or as much as you want)

Directions

Toss the 3 cups of fresh sweet corn, 2 cups of chopped roma tomatoes, 1/2 cup of chopped celery, 1/8 cup of fresh squeezed lemon juice and 1/4 of a chopped avocado in a medium sized bowl until the ingredients are evenly spread.

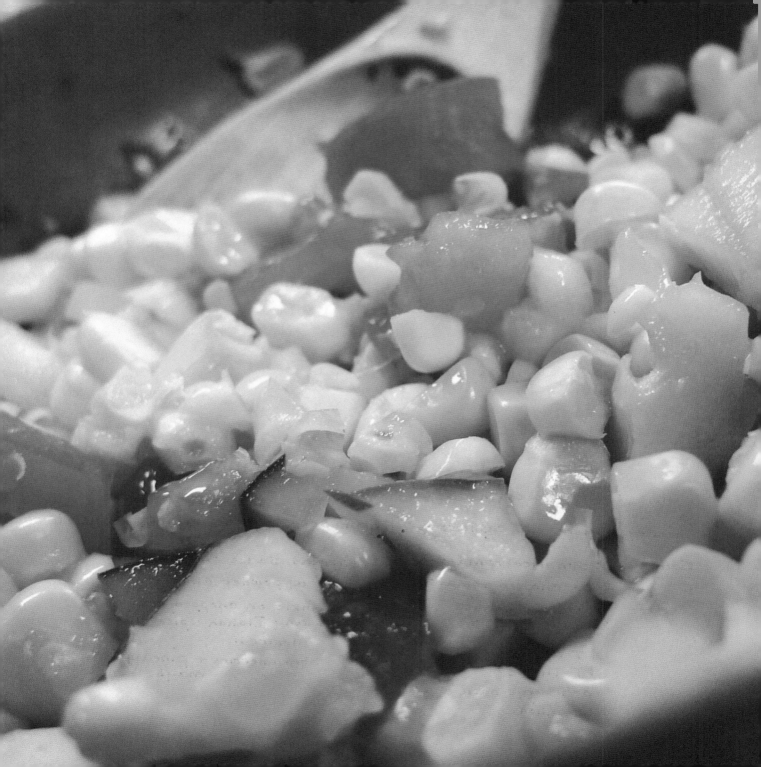

CUCUMBER TOMATO SLIDERS

Sometimes Something Simple Satisfies

Everyone who tries this dish is always pleasantly surprised. It is one of the easiest raw snacks to prepare. Not only does it look appetizing, but the taste is flavorful and refreshing.

Ingredients

16 Slices of Cucumber
16 Slices of Tomato
16 Pieces of Fresh Dill (1/2 Inch to 1 Inch)
4 Pitted Medjool Dates

Directions

Place the tomato slice on top of the cucumber slice. Cut the dates into 4 equal pieces each. Place one piece of date and one piece of dill on top. Serves 4 to 6 people.

Slice zucchini length wise

Cheeze (powdery) 2T cashews + 2T Hemp seeds - pulse in magic bullet

Sauce   1 c sundried tomatoes   spread sauce on zucchini
        2/3 c chopped tomatoes   top w/ powder cheeze
        1/3 c strawberries   sprinkle on chopped arugala
        2 T lemon juice   + any Italian spice as
        1 T Rosemary   desired.
        1 T Thyme   (strawberries + pineapple
        3-4 large basil leaves   maybe)
        2 scallions

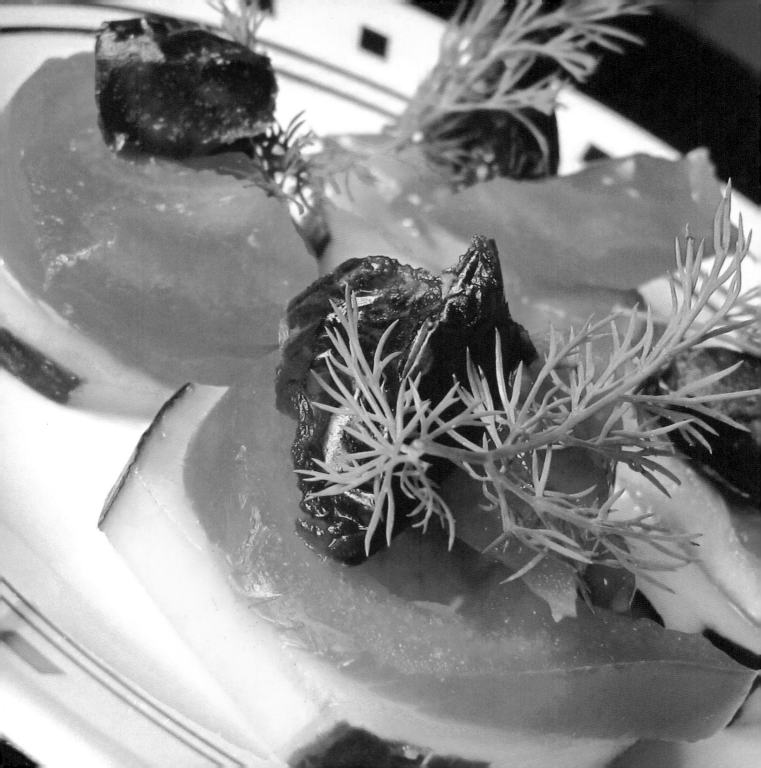

GINGER HORSERADISH SLAW

Ingredients

1/2 Cup Water
1/4 Cup Fresh Squeezed Lemon Juice
6 Pitted Medjool Dates
3 Quarter-Sized Medallions Horseradish Root
1 Quarter-Sized Medallion Fresh Ginger
3 Cups Jicama Sliced into Thin 2 Inch Long Pieces (You can use the shredding attachment on your food processor, if possible, to shred the jicama)
2 Cups Red Pepper Sliced into Thin 2 Inch Long Pieces
1 1/2 Cups Chopped Roma Tomatoes
1/3 Cup Chopped Scallions

Directions

Place 1/2 cup of water, 1/4 cup of fresh squeezed lemon juice, 6 pitted medjool dates, 3 quarter sized medallions of horseradish root (chopped into smaller pieces) and 1 quarter sized medallion of fresh ginger (chopped into smaller pieces) into the blender. Blend until creamy. Toss 3 cups of jicama, 2 cups of red pepper, 1 1/2 cups of chopped roma tomatoes and 1/3 cup of chopped scallions in a medium sized bowl. Add the dressing and toss until it is spread evenly. Serves 2 to 4 people.

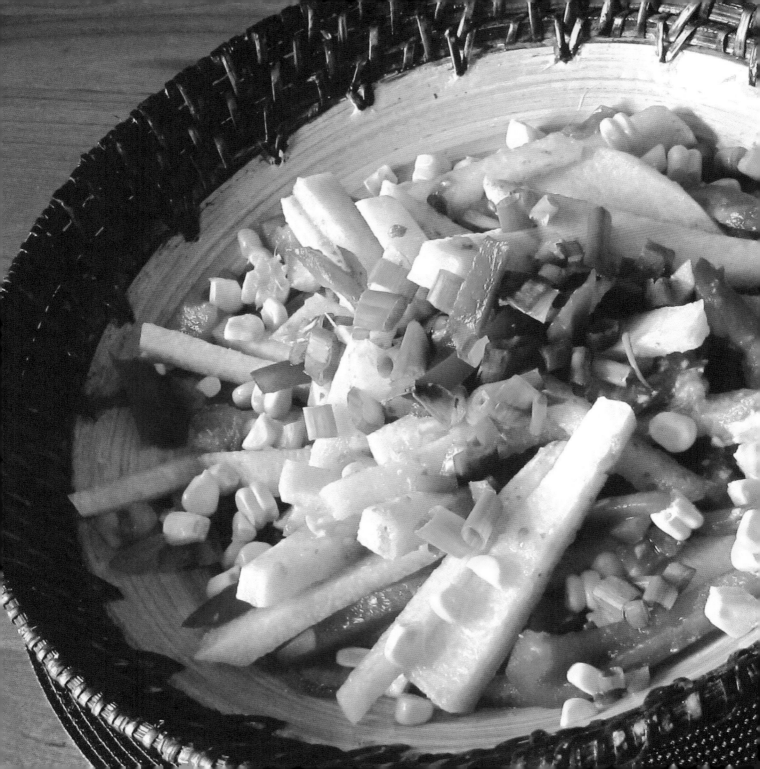

ZESTY AVOCADO POPPERS

Ingredients

1 3/4 Cups Chopped Fresh Pineapple
3/4 Cup Chopped Scallions
1/8 Cup Water (If needed)
2 Pitted Medjool Dates
1/2 Avocado
1/4 Cup Chopped Red Pepper
16 to 20 Cucumber Slices

Directions

Place 1 1/2 cups of pineapple, 1/2 cup of chopped scallions, 1/8 cup of water, 2 pitted medjool dates and 1/2 of an avocado into the blender. (You can also use a food processor and you will not need to use water. This will create a thicker texture.) Blend or process until creamy. Place a dollop of the zesty dip on a slice of cucumber and add a small piece of pineapple and red pepper. Sprinkle a few pieces of chopped scallion on top. Serves 4 to 6 people.

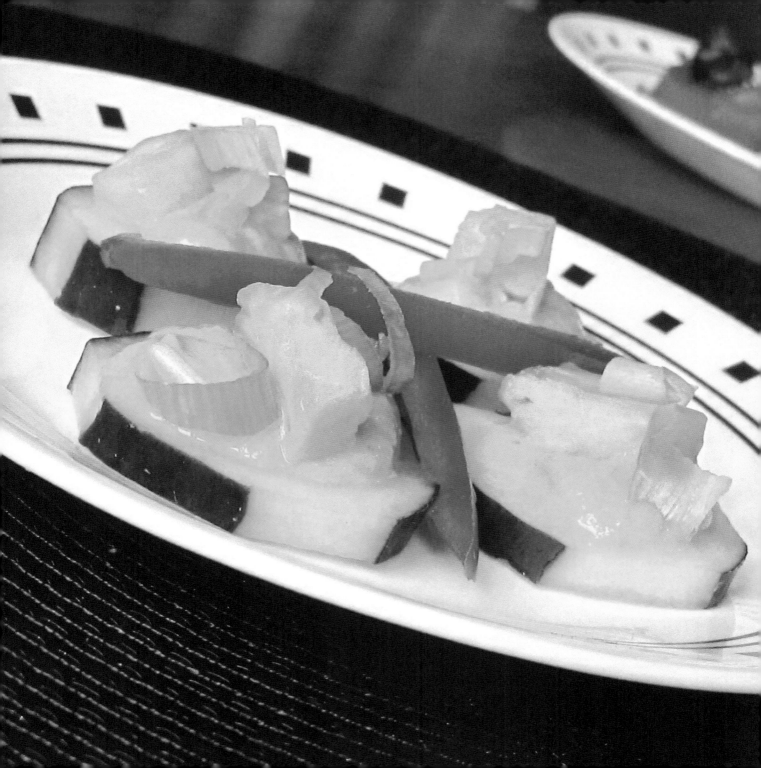

ENTREES

My favorite meal to have is zucchini pasta with a salad. It takes less than one minute to sprial cut a few zucchini or squash. If you make a few batches of sauce ahead of time you can have pasta a couple of times a week with minimal effort. Find or create your own favorite sauce. You can also add some spiral cut beet, carrot, or radish for a different color, texture, and taste.

Chili:
    2 c chopped tomatoes
    1/2 c peppers
    1/2 c orange juice
    1/2 c scallions
    1/4 c sundried tomatoes
    12 leaves oregano
    8 leaves sage
    1 c mushrooms

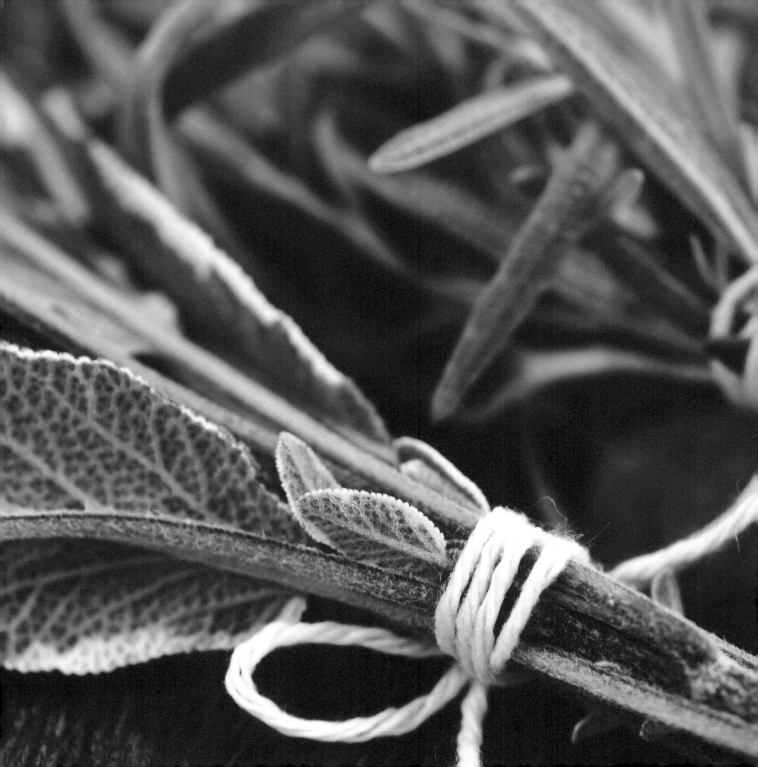

PASTA WITH TOMATO SAUCE

You can use the base from the tomato cherry soup or the zucchini noodle soup as a tomato sauce.

Ingredients

2 Cups Chopped Roma Tomatoes
2 to 4 Spiraled Zucchini
Tomato Sauce - Use Tomato Cherry Soup (page 20) or Zucchini Noodle Soup (page 22)

Vari add basil + sage

Directions

Place ingredients from either sauce option into blender and blend until creamy. Spiral cut the zucchini like spaghetti and dress with desired sauce and add 2 cups of chopped tomatoes on top. Serves 2 to 4 people.

Kristina's Epic Marinara Sauce/soup/Dressing

2 cartons cherry tomatoes
spinach
swiss chard stems - beet greens or celery
rosemary (not stems)
oregano
cilantro
dill
lemon

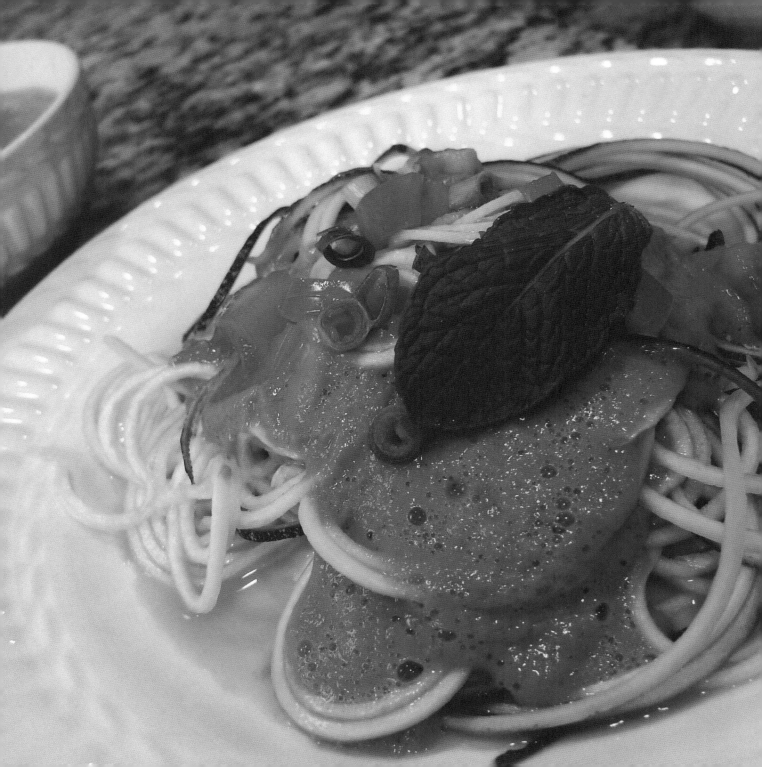

REFRESHING BASIL MINT PASTA

Ingredients

1 Cup Fresh Basil
1 Cup Fresh Mint
1/2 Cup Fresh Squeezed Lemon Juice
1/2 Cup water
3 Pitted Medjool Dates
1/4 Avocado
2 Cup Chopped Roma Tomatoes
3 to 4 Spiraled Zucchini

Spiralized cucumber
(let sit & drain water)

1 c almonds or pine nuts
2 c. basil
1 clove garlic
8 sun dried tom. soaked
12 peppercorns
sea salt
(very thick)

ICE CREAM:
1 frozen banana
10 frozen strawberries

Directions

Place 1 cup of fresh basil, 1 cup of fresh mint, 1/2 cup of fresh squeezed lemon juice, 1/2 cup of water, 3 pitted medjool dates and 1/4 of an avocado into the blender. Blend until creamy. Spiral cut the zucchini like spaghetti and place in a large bowl. Pour the pesto sauce on top and then add the 2 cups of chopped tomatoes for color. Toss if necessary. Serves 2 to 4 people.

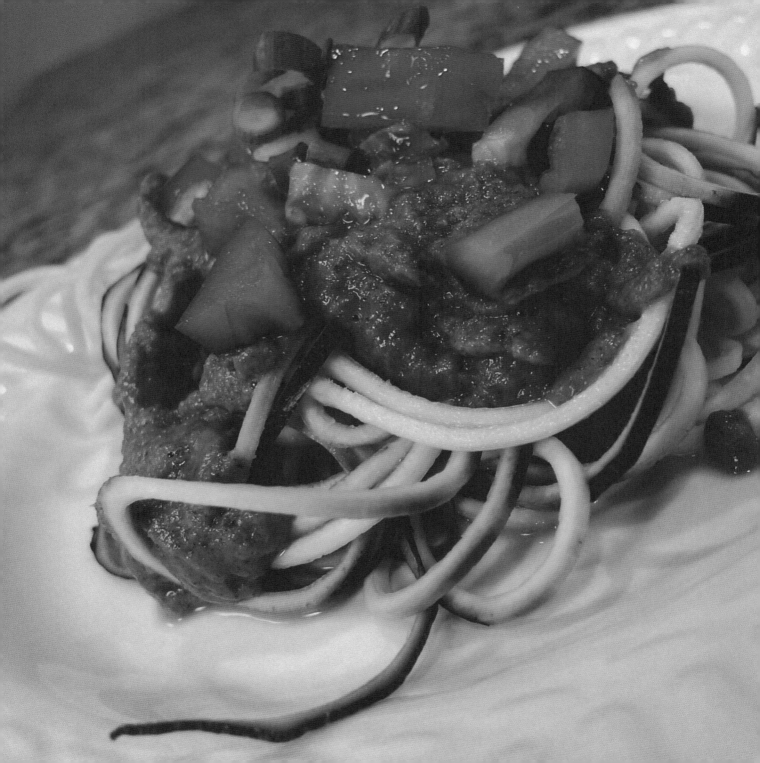

SAVORY ROMAINE TACOS

Ingredients

1 Cup Chopped Roma Tomatoes
1/2 Cup Chopped Scallions
1/4 Cup Frozen Pitted Cherries (Thawed)
5 Leaves of Fresh Cilantro
2 Leaves of Fresh Basil
1/2 Cup Fresh Sweet Corn off the Cob
1/4 Avocado Sliced or Chopped
6 to 8 Large Leaves of Romaine

Directions

Place 1/2 cup of chopped roma tomatoes, 1/4 cup of thawed cherries, 1/4 cup of chopped scallions, 5 leaves of cilantro and 2 leaves of basil into the blender. Blend until creamy. Spread about one tablespoon in each romaine leaf. Evenly distribute the 1/2 cup of fresh sweet corn, 1/2 cup of chopped roma tomatoes, 1/4 cup of chopped scallions, and 1/4 of an avocado between the 6 to 8 romaine leaves. Serves 2 to 4 people.

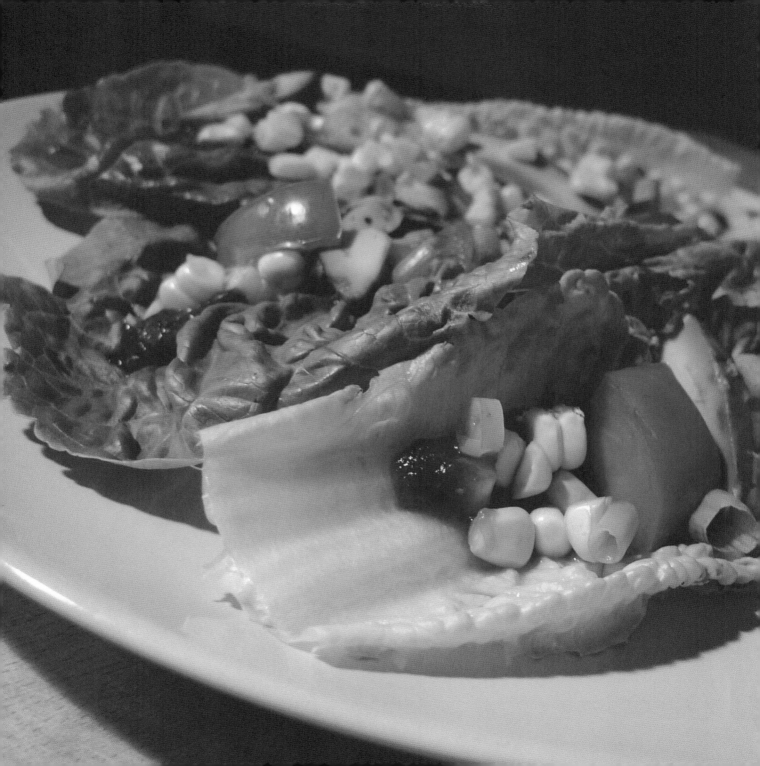

TABOULI STUFFED RED PEPPERS

Ingredients

1/2 Cup Fresh Squeezed Lemon Juice
3 Pitted Medjool Dates
2 Cups Chopped Heirloom Tomatoes
1 1/2 Cups Finely Chopped Fresh Parsley
1 1/2 Cups Chopped Cucumber
1/2 Cup Finely Chopped Fresh Cilantro
1 1/4 Cups Chopped Scallions
1/2 Teaspoon Hemp Seeds
2 to 4 Whole Red Peppers with Stem and Seeds Removed

Directions

Place 1/2 cup of fresh squeezed lemon, 1/4 cup of chopped scallions, and 3 pitted medjool dates into the blender. Blend until mostly smooth and add slightly more lemon juice if necessary. Toss in a large bowl 2 cups of chopped heirloom tomatoes, 1 1/2 cups of chopped cucumber, 1 1/2 cups of finely chopped fresh parsley, 1 cup of chopped scallions, 1/2 cup of finely chopped fresh cilantro and 1/4 teaspoon of hemp seeds. Pour the dressing into the large bowl and mix in with the other chopped ingredients until it is evenly spread throughout. Fill the hollowed red peppers with the tabouli and place whatever is left over on the side. Sprinkle the remaining 1/4 teaspoon of hemp seeds on top as a garnish. Serves 2 to 4 people.

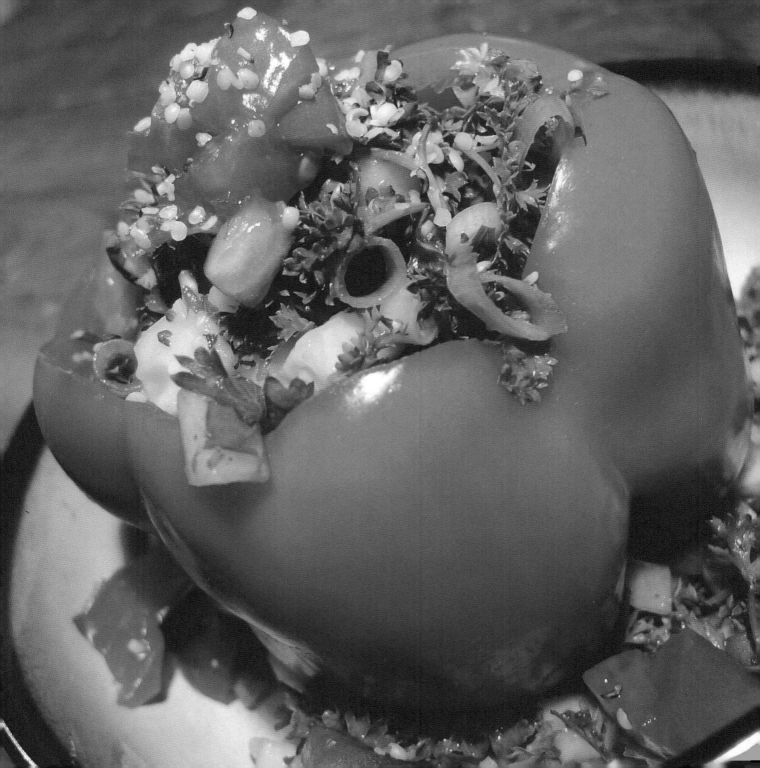

ZUCCHINI HEIRLOOM LASAGNA

Ingredients

1/2 Chopped Heirloom Tomatoes
1/4 Cup Frozen Pitted Cherries (Thawed)
1 Teaspoon Chopped Fresh Thyme
6 Leaves of Basil
8 Slices of Large Heirloom Tomatoes (Different Colors if Possible)
8 Thin Slices of Peeled Zucchini
1/4 Avocado Sliced in 8 Thin Pieces or Chopped

Directions

Place the 1/2 cup of chopped heirloom tomatoes, 1/4 cup of thawed cherries, 3/4 teaspoon of chopped fresh thyme, and 4 leaves of basil into the blender. Blend until creamy. Place 4 large slices of heirloom tomatoes on the center of the plate and spread with enough tomato sauce to slightly cover them. Lay 4 slices of zucchini over the tomatoes and spread with enough sauce to slightly cover them. Sprinkle some of the leftover thyme and lay 4 slices of avocado on top. Repeat in the same order with the next layers. Tomatoes, zucchini, sprinkle some thyme, then add avocado. Garnish with basil leaves. Serves 1 to 2 people.

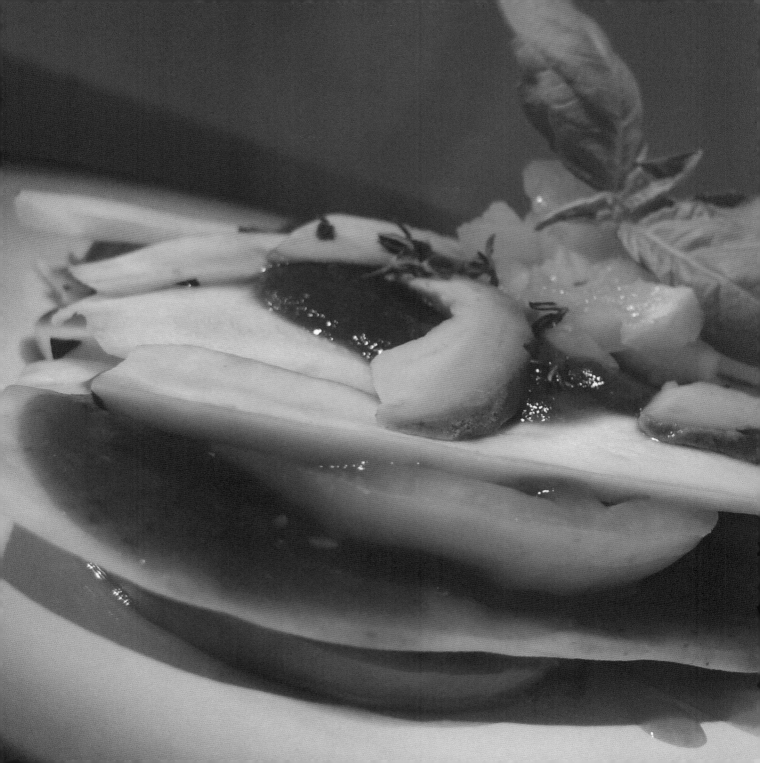

DESSERTS

Raw desserts made purely from fruit are the best! You can have dessert any time, guilt-free. After I eat a big salad I always have room for a perfectly ripe mango or a little piece of raw cherry pie. Many people say the best part about the raw food diet is the incredibly flavorful desserts . These dessert recipes are just a few simple ways to kick your fruit up a notch and satisfy your hungry eyes and tummies!

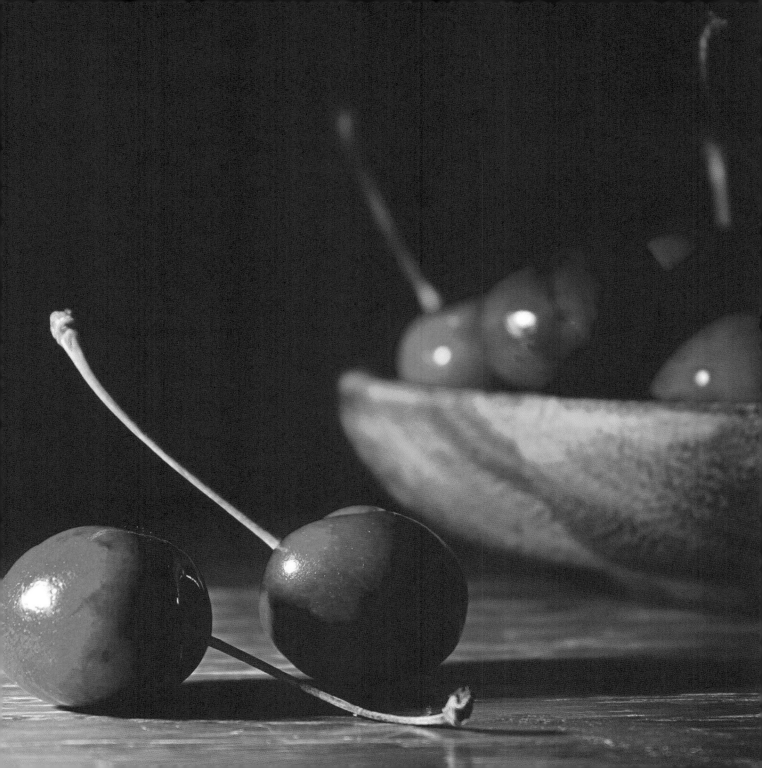

CHERRY PIE

This is the easiest cherry pie you will ever make.

Ingredients

1 1/2 Cups Pitted Chopped Medjool Dates
1/3 Cup Shredded Raw Coconut
1 to 1 1/2 Cups Frozen Cherries (Thawed)
4 to 6 Extra Cherries

Directions

Place 1 1/2 cups of chopped dates and only 1/4 cup of coconut in the food processor. Mix until the dates and coconut are spread evenly throughout. Press into the bottom of a 6 to 8 inch wide bowl or pie pan, or into 4 to 6 molds from a cupcake pan, to make the piecrust. Blend the 1 to 1 1/2 cups of thawed cherries until creamy. Pour the filling into the crust. Freeze for 2 to 3 hours. Wrap with plastic wrap if freezing overnight. When the filling is hard, garnish with a few cherries and the left over coconut. Serves 4 to 6 people.

Cherry parfait (Kristina)
Crust: dates + almonds pulsed
Layers cherry
dates
crust
Blended cherries + dates
Top: almonds + dates blended

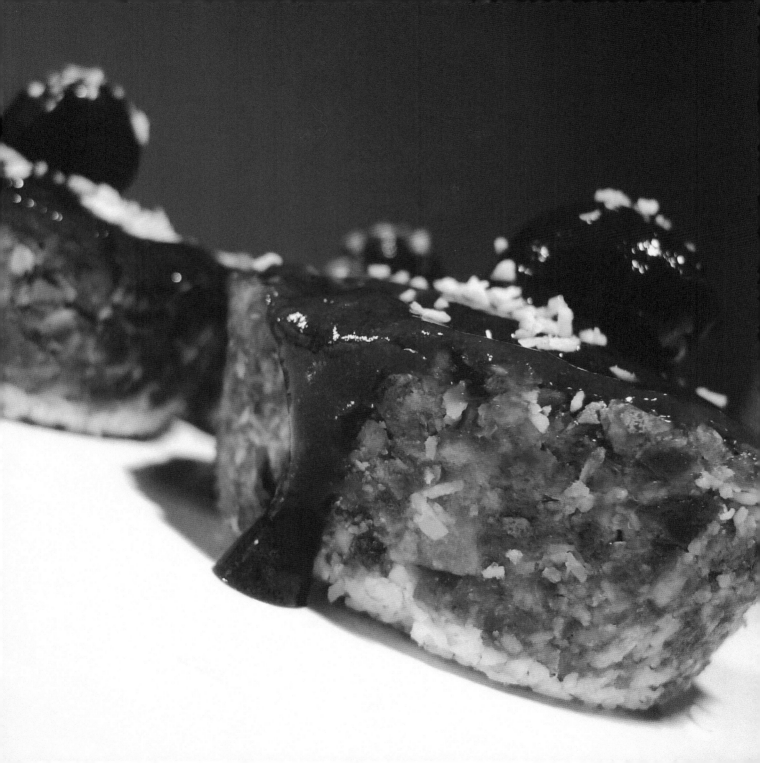

CINNAMON CARAMEL DIP WITH APPLES

Ingredients

1/2 to 3/4 Cup Water
Heaping 1/2 Teaspoon Ground Cinnamon
8 Pitted Medjool Dates
2 Apples of Any Variety

Directions

Place the 1/2 cup of water, heaping 1/2 teaspoon of cinnamon and chopped medjool dates into the blender. Blend until creamy (add more water if needed) and pour into a small bowl. Slice the apples into bite size pieces for dipping. Serves 4 to 6 people.

Apple Sauce Variation

Chop the apples and add them to the blender with the other ingredients. Blend until evenly mixed. Add 1/8 cup of fresh squeezed lemon juice if you want to store any leftovers in the fridge.

Butterscotch Dip
    8 dates
    1/2c dried mulberries soaked
    capful vanilla
    water

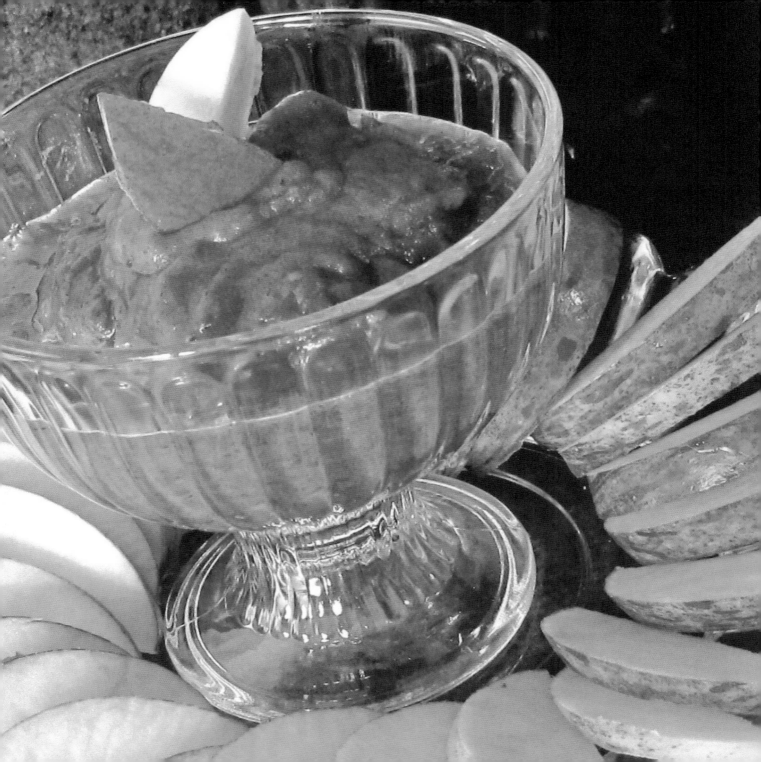

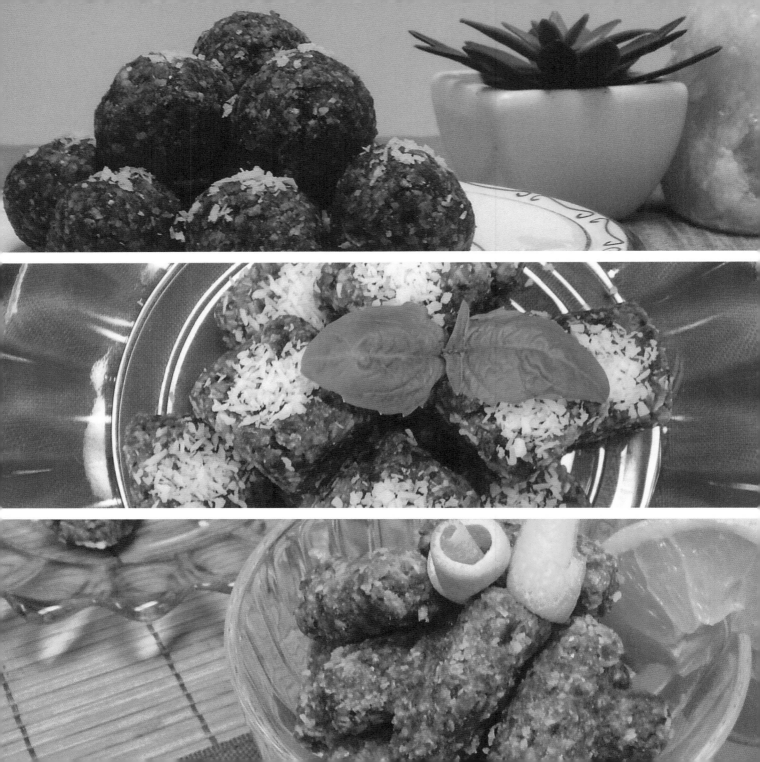

COCONUT DATE BITES

Three Variations - Serves 2 to 4 People

CINNAMON DOUGHNUT HOLES

Ingredients

3 Cups Pitted Medjool Dates
1/2 Cup Shredded Raw Coconut
3 Teaspoons Ground Cinnamon

AFTER DINNER MINTS

Ingredients

3 Cups Pitted Medjool Dates
1/2 Cup Shredded Raw Coconut
1/4 Cup Chopped Fresh Mint

ORANGE ROLLS

Ingredients

3 Cups Pitted Medjool Dates
1/2 Cup Shredded Raw Coconut
1/4 Cup Orange Zest

COCONUT DATE BITES

Directions

Place 3 cups of pitted medjool dates, 1/2 cup of shredded raw coconut, and either 3 teaspoons of ground cinnamon, 1/4 cup of chopped fresh mint, or 1/4 cup of orange zest into the food processor. Mix until the coconut, dates and other ingredients are even throughout.

Try Displaying The Coconut Date Bites in Different Ways

They all taste different, so why should they look the same? I like rolling the mix with cinnamon into balls because it makes me feel like I'm eating little doughnut holes. The mixture with mint looks pretty when you press them into tiny squares, sort of like a regular after dinner mint. It really feels like I am eating candy when I roll the mixture with orange into little log rolls.

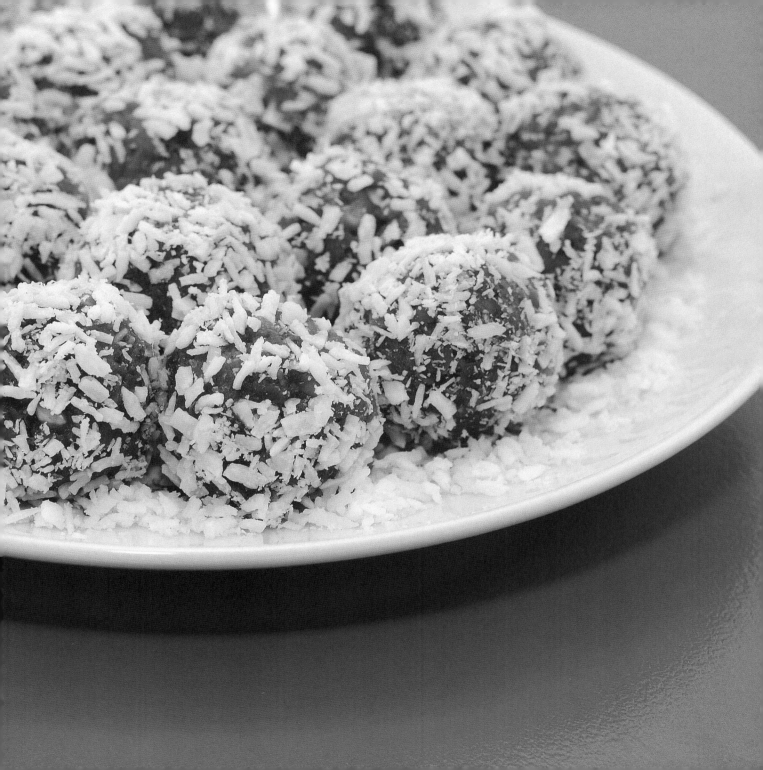

MANGO STRAWBERRY PIE

Ingredients

1 1/2 Cups Pitted Chopped Medjool Dates
1/3 Cup Shredded Raw Coconut
1/2 Teaspoon Ground Cinnamon
3/4 Cup of Chopped Fresh Mango
1/4 Cup Chopped Fresh Strawberries

Directions

Place 1 1/2 cups of chopped dates, only 1/4 cup of coconut and 1/2 teaspoon of cinnamon into the food processor. Mix until the dates, coconut, and cinnamon are spread evenly throughout. Press into the bottom of a 6 to 8 inch wide bowl or pie pan, or into 4 to 6 molds from a cupcake pan, to make the piecrust. Put a few pieces of chopped strawberry in the piecrust and save a few pieces to garnish the top. Blend the 3/4 cup of chopped mango until creamy and pour into the piecrust. Freeze for 2 to 3 hours. Wrap with plastic wrap if freezing overnight. When the filling is hard garnish with a few pieces of strawberry and left over coconut. Serves 4 to 6 people.

another filling Chocolate :
Blueberries, dates + 4 t raw cocoa powder
[no cinnamon in crust]

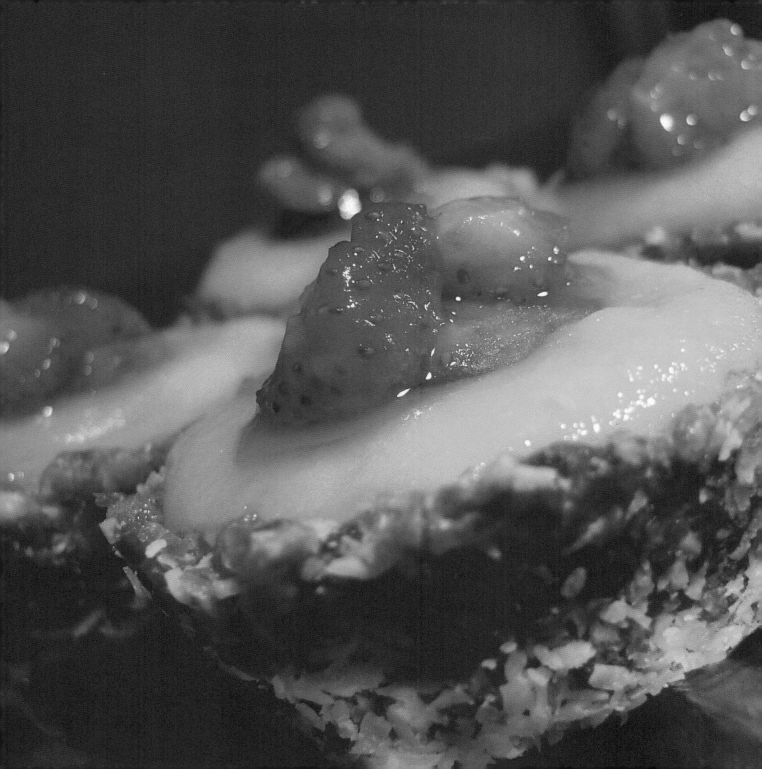

SMOOTHIES

There are endless, delicious combinations for fruit smoothies. There are thousands of fruits in the world so mix and match. When I first started eating raw food it was rare for me to make a smoothie. "Why would I want to drink my food, when I could eat it?", I thought. Then one day I made a cherry, date, and orange smoothie. Wow! I was amazed at how satisfying and convenient it was. Now, whenever I am out all day I make a giant smoothie and take it with me. It keeps me full and I don't have to think about what I am going to eat while I'm out. If you know you will be busy all day, make a couple of high calorie smoothies to keep yourself full. All of these smoothies should be made in a blender. Make sure to chop the ingredients to the appropriate size for your blender.

BANANA AND COMPANY

Ingredients

1 Cup Chopped Apple of Any Variety
1 Cup Chopped Frozen Bananas
1 Cup Peeled Chopped Orange Slices
1/4 Cup Pitted Chopped Medjool Dates

Bananas

Bananas are a staple food for many raw foodists. They have about 100 calories each and are loaded with vitamins , minerals, and electrolytes. They are also one of the cheapest and most available fruits. They are grown in 130 countries worldwide and are the fourth most widely consumed food in the world. Make bananas a staple food in your raw diet and you'll be living on easy street.

Chocolate Shake

2 bananas
1 apple
1 1/2 c water
2 dates
1 T chocolate (or carob)

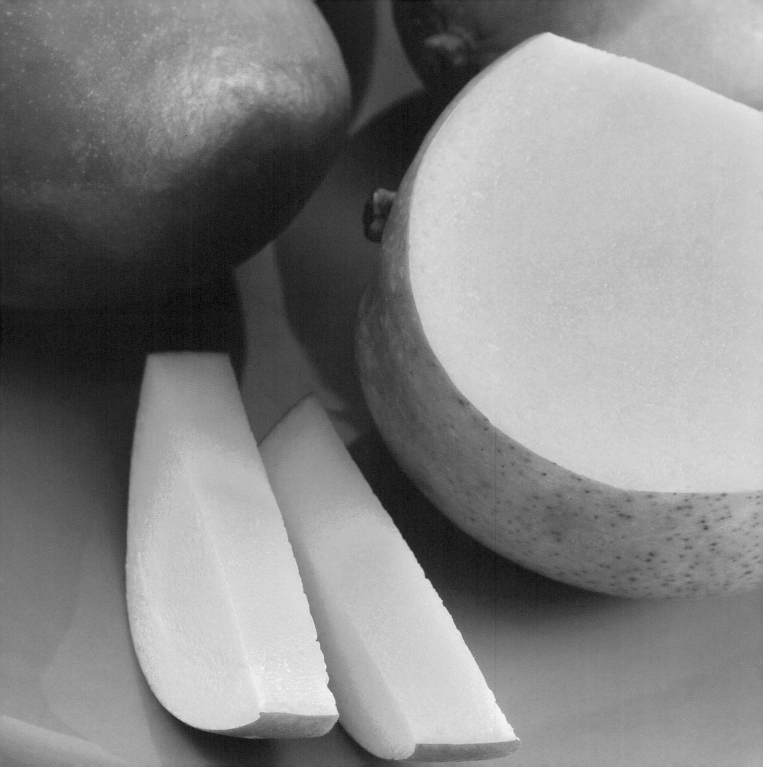

CHERRY BERRY

Ingredients

2 Cups Frozen Cherries
1 1/2 Cups Peeled Oranges
1/2 Cup Fresh or Frozen Strawberries
1/2 Cup Water
1/4 Cup Pitted Chopped Medjool Dates

Cherry Vanilla   2 cups
Coconut water from 1
2 dates
1/2 capful vanilla
1 c frozen cherries
5 Bananas

Cherries

Cherries are one of my favorite fruits to put in a smoothie and this is my favorite smoothie recipe. They are so creamy when you blend them up. They are also a great source of protien and antioxidants called anthocyanins, which is what makes them red. It helps detoxify the body, reduce inflammation, and lower uric acid in the joints and blood. Cherries are great for people who suffer from arthritis and gout.

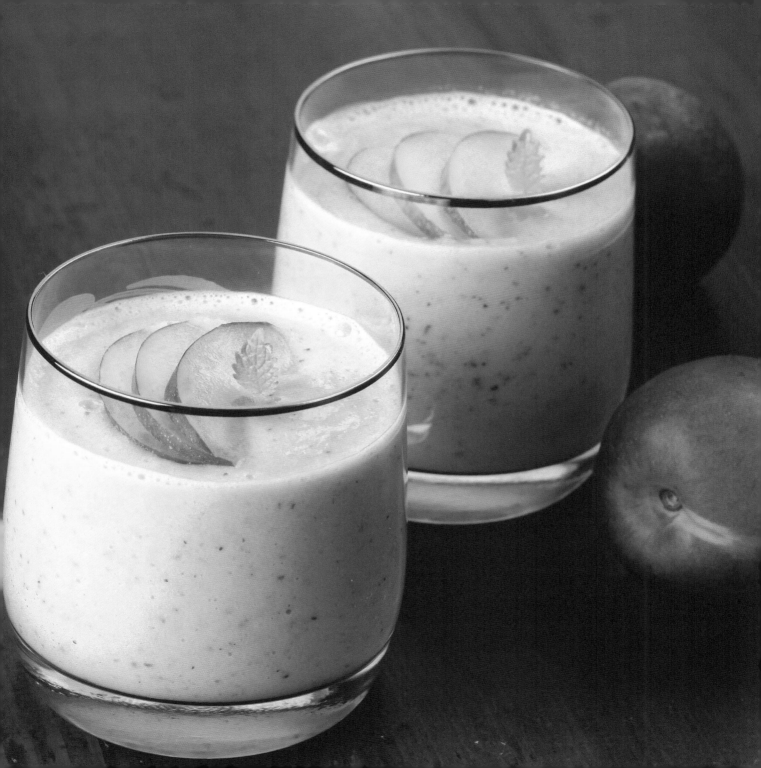

CINNAMON BANANA MILK

Ingredients

3 Cups Chopped Fresh or Frozen Bananas
1/2 Cup Water
1/4 Cup Chopped Medjool Dates
1 Teaspoon Ground Cinnamon

Yum!

This smoothie can be enjoyed frozen, at room temperature, or even warm. If you use fresh bananas and let your blender run for a minute or so, this smoothie will become slightly warm. It is great to drink if you have cold winters. You can add more cinnamon if you like or even some fresh vanilla bean if you have it.

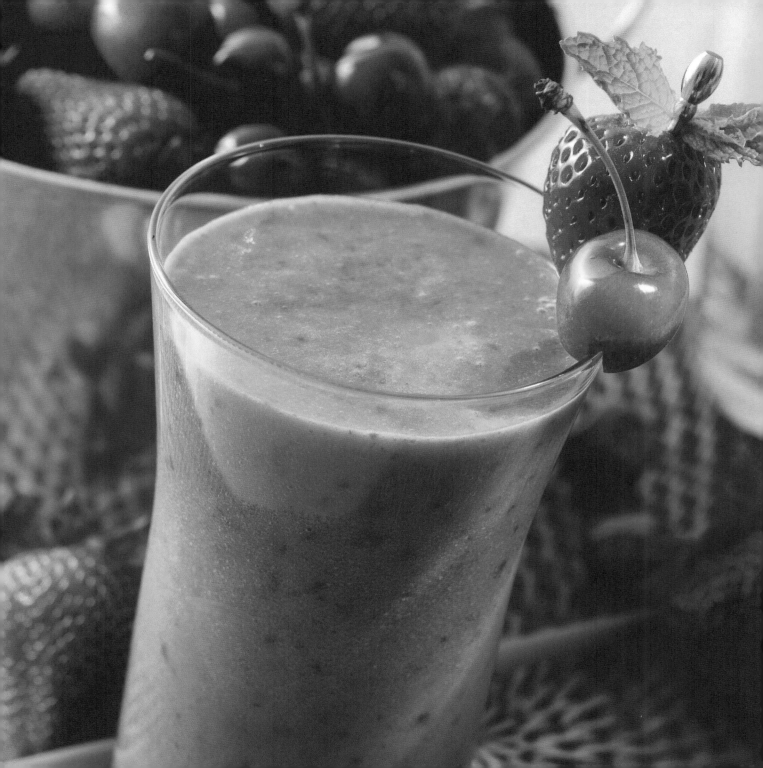

GREEN SMOOTHIE

Ingredients

2 Cups Chopped Frozen Bananas
1 Cup Chopped Greens (Spinach Blends Easily in Most Blenders)
3/4 Cup Chopped Apple
3/4 Cup Chopped Pear
1/2 Cup Water
1/4 Cup Pitted Chopped Medjool Dates

Arnold's Green Smoothie

This particular recipe for a green smoothie was created by Arnold Kauffman, the owner of Arnold's Way Raw Food Cafe. He came up with the recipe in 2007 after reading "Green for Life" by Victoria Boutenko. He says the green smoothie has boosted his business along with the health of his customers. Victoria Boutenko has a new book out called "Green Smoothie Revolution" which has inspired Arnold to create his own revolution. You can watch entertaining and educational videos of Arnold at www.youtube.com/arnoldsway.

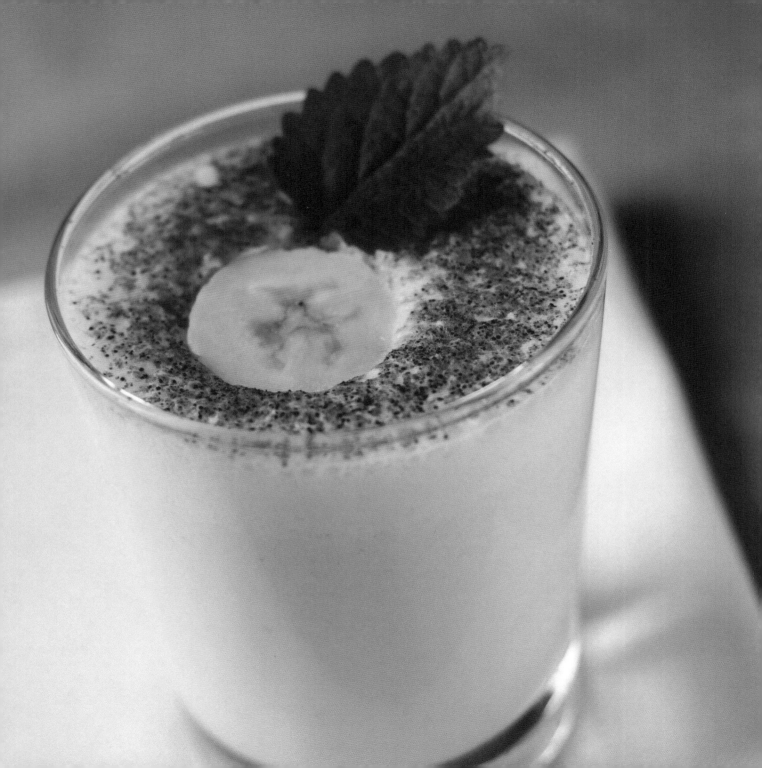

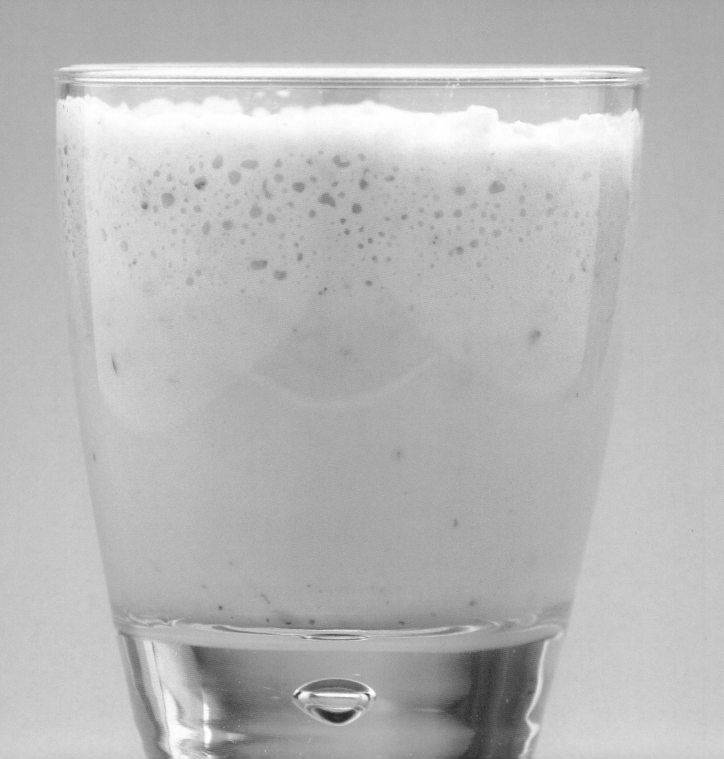

KIWI SURPRISE

Ingredients

1 1/2 Cups Peeled Chopped Fresh Mango
1 Cup Whole Fresh or Frozen Strawberries
1/3 Cup of Pitted Chopped Medjool Dates
1/2 Cup Peeled Chopped Kiwi
1/2 Cup Water

Surprise!

Everyone has probably had a kiwi strawberry smoothie, but have you ever had a kiwi strawberry mango smoothie? Okay, so what if you have! It is still delicious! This is a really refreshing summer smoothie. This combination of fruit also makes a beautiful and tasty fruit salad.

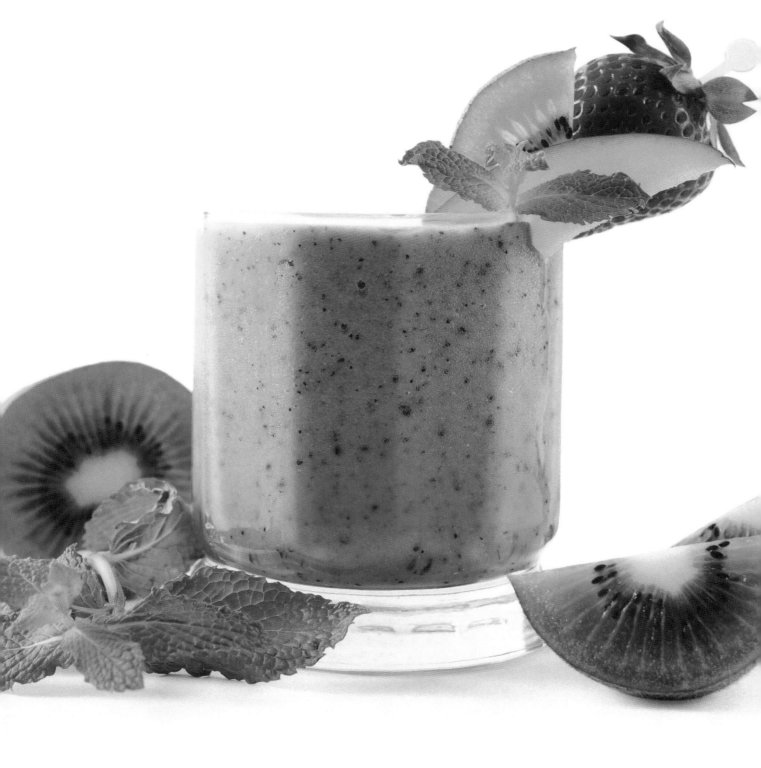

PAPAYA AND LIME

Ingredients

1 1/2 Cups Peeled Chopped Papaya
1 1/2 Cups Peeled Chopped Mango
1/2 Cup Water
1/4 Cup Fresh Squeezed Lime Juice
1/4 Cup Pitted Chopped Medjool Dates

Papaya

Papayas are great for digestion because they are approximately 91% water and contain a digestive enzyme called papin, which helps breakdown protein. It is effective in clearing skin when used topically or eaten. When I eat papaya regularly my skin glows. It is traditionally eaten with lime juice. For breakfast try cutting up some papaya and sprinkling lime juice on top. Don't forget to save some for your face!

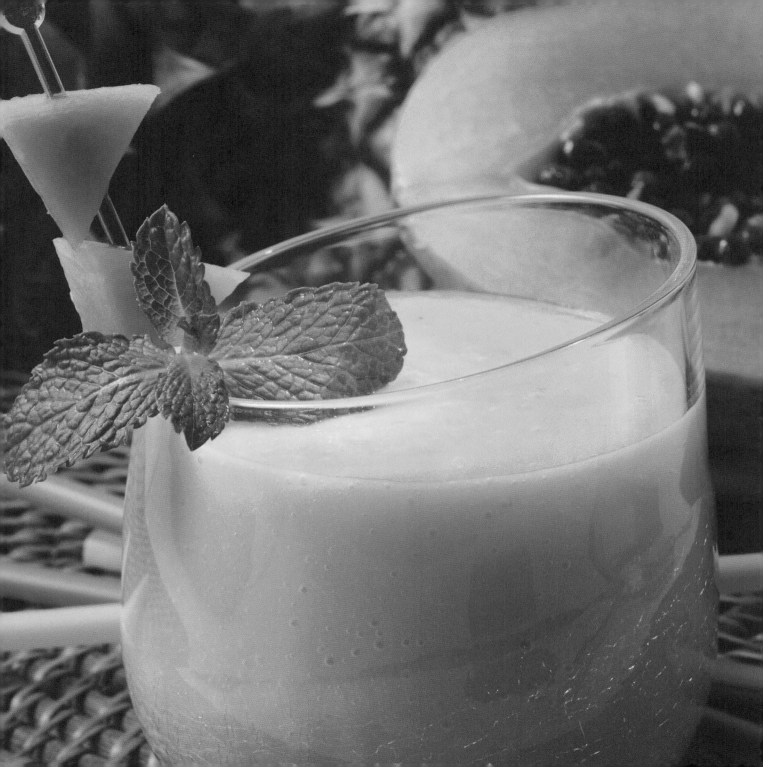

TROPICAL BERRY

Raw Winter Smoothie:
6 c orange juice
1 1/2 c. frozen berries
or pineapple

Ingredients

1 Cup Peeled Chopped Fresh Mango
1 Cup Peeled Chopped Orange Slices
1 Cup Whole Fresh or Frozen Strawberries
1/2 Cup Water
1/3 Cup Pitted Chopped Medjool Dates

Strawberries

Did you know that there are over 600 varieties of strawberries and that it is considered the most popular fruit in the world? They are an all around amazing fruit. Low in calories and high in water content, nutrients, and taste. They have similar health benefits to cherries because strawberries contain anthocyanin as well.

Var:
1 c. orange juice
pineapple.
strawberries
pink lady apples

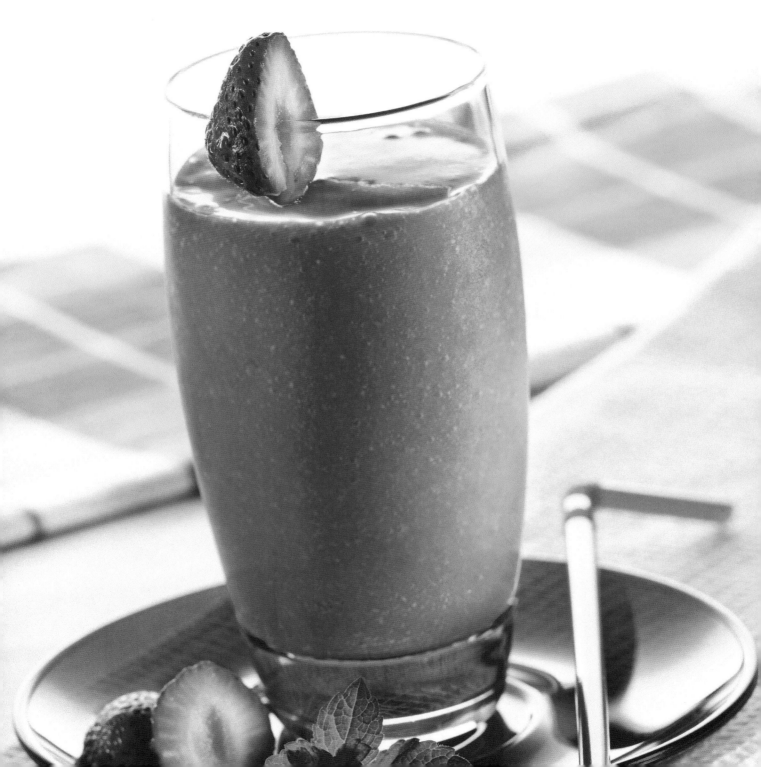

LIVING CONSCIOUSLY

We are on this Earth to learn, grow, and enjoy the experience of life. We are responsible for taking care of our minds and bodies. If we do not provide ourselves with proper nutrition, exercise, and a healthy environment, then we are greatly reducing our personal potential in more ways than we know. Developing healthy relationships with people and food will help you stay on track with your personal goals.

EATING CONSCIOUSLY

Eating consciously means giving your food choices a little thought. What am I supporting? Does what I'm supporting, support me? Is it sustainable? Am I taking away the freedom of life from another being? Is what I'm doing working for me? You should feel confident about your answers to these questions. If you don't, you may need to make some changes.

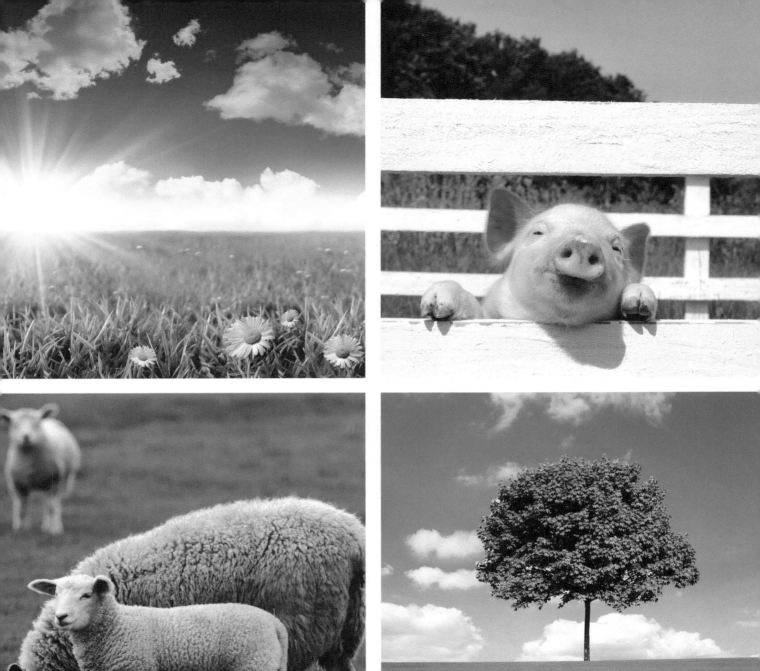

RECOMMENDED BOOKS & MOVIES
I Recommend That You Read:

80/10/10
By Dr. Douglas Graham

Your Natural Diet
By David Klein and T.C. Fry

The Food Revolution
By John Robbins

The World Peace Diet
By Will Tuttle

I Recommend That You Watch:

Peaceable Kingdom
By James LaVeck and Jenny Stein

Earthlings
By Shaun Monson

[NOT EASY]
No Tatoes
Celery Root
   water
   Cashews
      garlic
      white pepper
      miso
      salt
      onion powder
   Nut. yeast
      chives (mix in by hand)

Gravy
   olive oil
or poechini mushrooms
   oyster
   nuts
   nama shoyu
   nut. yeast
   garlic
   poultry seasoning
   onion

Dressing or Pasta Sauce:

1. 1 c peaches (or mango)   Blend
   cherry tomatoes

2. 3 T tahini
   1/4 c water   blend with spoon adding a little
                  water at a time.

Pad Thai

1/2 c orange juice
1/3 c coconut meat
1/3 c scallions
2 T lemon juice
sage
1/4 inch ginger
1 1/2 T tahini

Noodles:
1/2 c spiralized carrot
1/2 pepper (red, orange or yellow)
3 1/2 zucchini

Make noodles 1st
add lemon juice to soften

Pour on sauce & let sit
15 minutes

Pie (made with mame sapote)

Crust: 10 dates + 3 t shredded coconut   Food Processor
       press into bottom of small spring form pan

Filling - sweet potato + fruit (squash etc)
       5 t chocolate
       6 dates
       1/4 t cinnamon

Freeze 1 hour or frig 3-4 hours

Mango Chutney

In Processor:

    2 c chopped tomato
    2 c mango
    3/4 c scallion (green only)
    2 dates
    2 T lemon juice

Pulse for salsa

Simple dressing: 1 c mango, 3-4 dates, 1 c water as needed.

Mango Thai : 1 c mango
              1/4 inch medallion of ginger
              1/8 c. cashews
              1/4 c. scallions
              3-4 dates
              water as needed

Oatmeal:
    4 c chopped apple
    2 dates   [pulse]
    1/4 c cashews

Top with frozen banana whip

[can make with mango + pineapple] [cashews opt]

Chili   Chopped Veg in Bowl   tomatoes, avocado
                              - mushrooms, broccoli -anything

    Sauce   2 c. chopped tomatoes
            1/2 c peppers
            1/2 c orange juice
            1/2 c scallions
            1/4 c sundried tomatoes
            12 leaves oregano
            8 "   sage
            1/4 avocado

More Smoothies

2 oranges
2 Lg. carrots
1 inch ginger
Little water + ice

2 carrots
1 apple
spinach
1 T grated ginger
6 oz water

3 bananas
1 mango
8 strawberries
3 c dandelion greens
1 head leaf lettuce
hemp seeds
8 oz. water

Veggie Dip

1 c zucchini
1 c scallion (green)
2 T dill
1/4 c hemp seeds
1/2 c lemon juice
1 1/2 T Rosemary
   Blend

1 c. blueberries
2 apples
1 peeled beet   (rub hands w/ veg. oil)
1 carrot
3 leaves kale

Salad Dressing   the Raw Food Effect.com

1 Red bell pepper
1 whole orange
4 dates
a little water

[Kristina]

Salad

Salad — pulse kale + chopped zucchini

Dressing — nectarines + strawberries

Top with blueberries

Avacado, Orange + Jicama with Coriander Dressing

Dressing: 1/3 c. oj.
3 T lime juice
(1 T olive oil)
1 t. coriander seeds crushed
1 clove garlic minced
Blend 10 sec
add 2 T cilantro leaves
+ pinch of salt + pepper

Salad:
2 large oranges (1 cup)
1/4 small jicama cubed or matchsticked
6 c. butter lettuce
1 avocado sliced

Raw Vegan Burgers

1 1/2 c sun dried tomatoes soaked 30 min. Pat dry
3/4 c sunflower seeds   "   "   "   "   "
2 c carrots or 2 c carrot pulp from juicing
1/2 c green onion (green only)
1/8 t. mustard seed
Squeeze of Lime

Made in the USA
Charleston, SC
29 April 2012